PEDIATRIC ESSENTIALS

A Guide to Sub-specialty Diagnosis

Brian Temple, M.D.

Renegade Medical Books

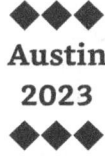

Austin

2023

Medical Disclaimer

The information provided in this infant medical book is for educational purposes only and is not intended to replace professional medical advice, diagnosis, or treatment. Always consult with a qualified healthcare provider or pediatrician regarding any specific medical questions or concerns you may have regarding your baby's health.

The content presented in this book is based on general knowledge and recommendations available up to September 2021. Medical practices, guidelines, and research may evolve over time, and new information may emerge that could affect the accuracy or applicability of the information provided herein. Therefore, it is essential to stay updated with current medical literature and consult trusted healthcare professionals for the most recent and appropriate advice.

The authors, publishers, and distributors of this book do not assume any liability for any direct, indirect, consequential, or incidental damages that may arise from the use of the information contained within. Any reliance on the information provided in this book is at the reader's own risk.

While every effort has been made to ensure the accuracy and completeness of the information presented, errors or omissions may occur. The authors, publishers, and distributors of this book shall not be held responsible for any inaccuracies or omissions or for any consequences arising from the use of the information provided.

By reading this book, you acknowledge and agree to the above disclaimer and understand that the information provided should not be used as a substitute for professional medical advice. Always consult with a qualified healthcare provider or pediatrician for personalized guidance and recommendations regarding your baby's health and well-being.

I dedicate this book and my life to my family

TABLE OF CONTENTS

Introduction
Chapter 1: Cardiology
Chapter 2: Gastroenterology
Chapter 3: Endocrinology
Chapter 4: Neurology
Chapter 5: Hematology and Oncology
Chapter 6: Pulmonology
Chapter 7: Rheumatology
Chapter 8: Nephrology
Chapter 9: Infectious Disease
Chapter 10: Dermatology
Chapter 11: Developmental and Behavioral
Chapter 12: Urology
Chapter 13: Ophthalmology
Chapter 14: Genetics
Chapter 15: Otolaryngology
Chapter 16: Allergy and Immunology
Chapter 17: Pathology
Chapter 18: Physical Medicine and Rehabilitation
Chapter 19: Emergency Medicine
Chapter 20: Neonatology
Chapter 21: Psychiatry
Conclusion

INTRODUCTION

Pediatric medicine is the branch of medicine that deals with the medical care of infants, children, and adolescents, from birth up to 18 years of age. Pediatric medicine is unique in that it requires not only specialized medical knowledge but also a unique understanding of child development, psychology, and family dynamics. Pediatricians not only diagnose and treat childhood illnesses and injuries but also provide preventive care, monitor growth and development, and offer guidance and support to families throughout the various stages of childhood.

One of the primary goals of pediatric medicine is to promote the health and well-being of children and adolescents. Pediatricians play a crucial role in ensuring that children receive the necessary vaccinations, screenings, and developmental assessments to help prevent disease and detect any potential problems early on. They also provide education and counseling to families on healthy lifestyle choices, such as proper nutrition, exercise, and safety practices.

In addition to primary care, pediatric medicine also includes specialized care for children with chronic medical conditions, developmental disabilities, and mental health issues. Pediatricians work closely with other healthcare providers, such as pediatric surgeons, neonatologists, and a multitude of other pediatric subspecialists, to provide comprehensive care to children with complex medical needs.

In this book, the most frequently encountered pediatric medical issues will be discussed within the specific specialty that they fall under.

Pediatric Specialties

Pediatric medicine is a branch of medicine that specializes in the medical care of infants, children, and adolescents. Within the field of pediatric medicine, there are several sub-specialties that focus on specific areas of care. Here are some of the most common pediatric specialties:

1.   Cardiology: This specialty focuses on the diagnosis and treatment of heart and cardiovascular problems in children.
2.   Gastroenterology: This specialty focuses on the diagnosis and treatment of digestive system disorders in children, including conditions such as Crohn's disease, ulcerative colitis, and celiac disease.
3.   Endocrinology: This specialty focuses on the diagnosis and treatment of hormonal disorders in children, including diabetes, growth disorders, and thyroid problems.
4.   Neurology: This specialty focuses on the diagnosis and treatment of neurological disorders in children, including epilepsy, cerebral palsy, and developmental delays.
5.   Oncology: This specialty focuses on the diagnosis and treatment of cancer in children, including leukemia, lymphoma, and brain tumors.
6.   Pulmonology: This specialty focuses on the diagnosis and treatment of respiratory disorders in children, including asthma, cystic fibrosis, and bronchitis.
7.   Rheumatology: This specialty focuses on the diagnosis and treatment of autoimmune and inflammatory disorders in children, including juvenile idiopathic arthritis and lupus.

8.   Nephrology: This specialty focuses on the diagnosis and treatment of kidney and urinary tract disorders in children, including kidney disease and urinary tract infections.

9.   Infectious disease: This specialty focuses on the diagnosis and treatment of infectious diseases in children, including measles, mumps, rubella, and chickenpox.

10. Dermatology is a specialty that focuses on the diagnosis and treatment of skin, hair, and nail conditions in children.

11. Developmental and behavioral pediatrics: This specialty focuses on the diagnosis and treatment of developmental and behavioral disorders in children, including ADHD, autism, and learning disabilities.

12. Urology is a surgical subspecialty that focuses on the diagnosis and treatment of urological conditions in children.

13. Ophthalmology is a medical and surgical subspecialty that deals with eye disorders and vision problems in children.

14. Genetics: pediatric geneticists, diagnose and manage genetic conditions in children.

15. Otolaryngology, also known as pediatric ENT (ear, nose, and throat) is a specialized field of medicine that focuses on the diagnosis and treatment of disorders related to the head and neck in children.

16. Allergy and Immunology is a specialized field of medicine that focuses on the diagnosis and treatment of allergies and immune system disorders in children.

17. Pathology: Pediatric pathology is a specialized field of medicine that focuses on the diagnosis of diseases and conditions that affect children from infancy to adolescence.

18. Physical Medicine and Rehabilitation:(PM&R) focuses on the diagnosis, treatment, and management of children

with physical and functional disabilities resulting from congenital conditions, developmental disorders, injuries, or illnesses.

19. Pediatric Emergency Medicine: A medical specialty that focuses on the diagnosis, treatment, and management of acutely ill or injured children.

20. Neonatology: a subspecialty that focuses on the care of newborn infants, particularly those who are premature, critically ill, or have medical or surgical conditions that require specialized care.

21. Psychiatry: A specialized field of medicine that focuses on the diagnosis and treatment of mental health disorders in children and adolescents.

CHAPTER 1

Cardiology

Pediatric cardiology is a medical specialty that deals with the diagnosis and treatment of heart problems in infants, children, and adolescents. Some of the common diagnoses that are treated by pediatric cardiologists include:

Congenital heart defects: These are heart problems that are present at birth, and can range from mild defects that may not require treatment to severe defects that require surgery or other interventions.

a. Atrial septal defect (ASD): This is a hole in the wall (septum) that separates the upper chambers of the heart.
b. Ventricular septal defect (VSD): This is a hole in the wall (septum) that separates the lower chambers of the heart.
c. Patent ductus arteriosus (PDA): This is a condition where a blood vessel, called the ductus arteriosus, fails to close after birth, which causes blood to flow between the two main arteries.
d. Tetralogy of Fallot (TOF): This is a combination of four heart defects that can lead to reduced blood flow to the body.
e. Coarctation of the aorta: This is a narrowing of the aorta, the major blood vessel that carries

oxygen-rich blood from the heart to the body.

f. Transposition of the great vessels: This is a defect where the aorta and pulmonary artery are switched, which can cause difficulty in getting enough oxygen to the body.

g. Hypoplastic left heart syndrome (HLHS): This is a rare condition in which the left side of the heart is underdeveloped and unable to pump enough blood to the body.

h. Pulmonary stenosis: This is a narrowing of the pulmonary valve, which can make it difficult for blood to flow from the heart to the lungs.

i. Aortic stenosis: This is a narrowing of the aortic valve, which can make it difficult for blood to flow from the heart to the body.

j. Congenital heart block: A rare congenital birth defect that affects the electrical system of the heart.

k. Pediatric arrhythmias are abnormal heart rhythms that occur in children

l. Cardiomyopathy: This is a condition in which the heart muscle becomes enlarged, thickened, or stiff, and can lead to heart failure or other complications.

m. Rheumatic fever: This is a complication of strep throat that can cause inflammation and damage to the heart valves.

n. Kawasaki disease: This is a condition that can cause inflammation of the blood vessels throughout the body, including the coronary arteries, and can lead to heart damage.

o. Pulmonary hypertension: This is a condition in which the blood vessels in the lungs become narrow, making it harder for blood to flow through them.

p. Syncope: This is a temporary loss of

consciousness or fainting, which can be caused by a variety of heart problems.

q. Chest pain: This is a common complaint in children, and can be caused by a variety of conditions including heart problems.

r. Hypertension: This is high blood pressure, which can be caused by a variety of factors including obesity, kidney problems, or certain medications.

s. Lipid disorders: These are disorders of cholesterol and other fats in the blood, which can increase the risk of heart disease.

Atrial Septal Defect (ASD)

Atrial septal defect (ASD) is a congenital heart defect that occurs when there is a hole in the wall (septum) that separates the upper chambers of the heart.

Diagnosis:

- Echocardiogram (a type of ultrasound that uses sound waves to create images of the heart) which can be done as early as the first days of life.
- Other diagnostic tools may include a chest x-ray, electrocardiogram (ECG), and a cardiac catheterization (a procedure that uses a thin tube to look inside the heart and blood vessels).

Treatment:

- Determined on the size of the defect, the symptoms it causes, and the child's overall health.

- Smaller defects may not require treatment and may close on their own over time.
- Larger defects may require surgery to repair the hole, which can be done through open heart surgery or by a catheter-based procedure.

Prognosis:

- Prognosis dependent on the size of the defect, the symptoms it causes, and the overall health of the child.
- Smaller defects may not cause any symptoms and may close on their own over time, resulting in a good prognosis.
- Larger defects may cause symptoms such as shortness of breath, fatigue, and heart failure and may require surgery. The prognosis after surgery is generally good, but depends on the child's overall health and the specific circumstances of the surgery.

Signs and symptoms: The signs and symptoms of ASD in a newborn can vary depending on the size of the hole and the overall health of the baby. Some newborns with an ASD may have no signs or symptoms, while others may have severe symptoms. Here are some common signs and symptoms of ASD in newborns:

1. Rapid breathing or difficulty breathing: Newborns with an ASD may have rapid breathing or difficulty breathing due to the extra workload on the heart.
2. Fatigue or poor feeding: Newborns with an ASD may tire easily and have trouble feeding due to the extra workload on the heart.
3. Persistent or recurrent lung infections: Newborns with an ASD may be more susceptible to lung infections due to the extra blood flow to the lungs.

4. Heart murmur: A heart murmur is an abnormal sound heard during a heartbeat, which can be caused by the extra blood flow through the hole in the septum.

5. Swelling of the legs, feet or abdomen: Newborns with an ASD may have swelling in their legs, feet, or abdomen due to the extra blood flow to the lungs and the increased pressure in the heart.

6. Bluish skin (cyanosis): Newborns with an ASD may have bluish skin due to the lack of oxygen in the blood.

Ventricular Septal Defect (VSD)

Ventricular septal defect (VSD) is a congenital heart defect that occurs when there is a hole in the wall (septum) that separates the lower chambers of the heart.

Signs and symptoms:

- Some newborns with a VSD may have no signs or symptoms, while others may have severe symptoms, such as:
- Rapid breathing or difficulty breathing
- Fatigue or poor feeding
- Persistent or recurrent lung infections
- Heart murmur
- Swelling of the legs, feet, or abdomen
- Bluish skin (cyanosis)

Diagnosis:

- The most common way to diagnose a VSD is through an echocardiogram (a type of ultrasound that uses sound waves to create images of the heart) which can be done as early as the first days of life.
- Other diagnostic tools may include a chest x-ray,

electrocardiogram (ECG), and a cardiac catheterization (a procedure that uses a thin tube to look inside the heart and blood vessels).

Treatment:

- Treatment for a VSD depends on the size of the defect, the symptoms it causes, and the child's overall health.
- Smaller defects may not require treatment and may close on their own over time.
- Larger defects may require surgery to repair the hole, which can be done through open heart surgery or by a catheter-based procedure.

Prognosis:

- VSD prognosis depends on the size of the defect, the symptoms it causes, and the overall health of the child.
- Smaller defects may not cause any symptoms and may close on their own over time, resulting in a good prognosis.
- Larger defects may cause symptoms such as shortness of breath, fatigue, and heart failure and may require surgery. The prognosis after surgery is generally good, but depends on the child's overall health and the specific circumstances of the surgery.

Patent Ductus Arteriosus (PDA)

Patent ductus arteriosus (PDA) is a congenital heart defect that occurs when the ductus arteriosus, a blood vessel that connects the aorta and the pulmonary artery, fails to close after birth.

Signs and symptoms:

- Some newborns have no signs or symptoms, while others may have severe symptoms, such as:
- Rapid breathing or difficulty breathing
- Fatigue or poor feeding
- Persistent or recurrent lung infections
- Heart murmur
- Swelling of the legs, feet, or abdomen
- Bluish skin (cyanosis)

Diagnosis:

- The most common way to diagnose PDA is through an echocardiogram (a type of ultrasound that uses sound waves to create images of the heart) which can be done as early as the first days of life.
- Other diagnostic tools may include a chest x-ray, electrocardiogram (ECG), and a cardiac catheterization (a procedure that uses a thin tube to look inside the heart and blood vessels).

Treatment:

- The size of the defect, the symptoms it causes, and the child's overall health will determine the treatment for PDA
- Smaller defects may not require treatment and may close on their own over time.
- Larger defects may require surgery to repair the ductus arteriosus, which can be done through open heart surgery

or by a catheter-based procedure.
- Medications such as ibuprofen can be used to close the ductus arteriosus.

Prognosis:

- PDA prognosis depends on the size of the defect, the symptoms it causes, and the overall health of the child.
- Smaller defects may not cause any symptoms and may close on their own over time, resulting in a good prognosis.
- Larger defects may cause symptoms such as shortness of breath, fatigue, and heart failure and may require surgery. The prognosis after surgery is generally good, but depends on the child's overall health and the specific circumstances of the surgery.

Tetralogy of Fallot (TOF)

Tetralogy of Fallot (TOF) is a congenital heart defect that is a combination of four heart defects that can lead to reduced blood flow to the body. These defects include:

- A ventricular septal defect (VSD), which is a hole in the wall that separates the lower chambers of the heart
- Obstruction of the outflow of blood from the right ventricle, which causes the right ventricle to become enlarged
- An overriding aorta, which means that the aorta is located above both ventricles instead of just the left one
- Right ventricular hypertrophy, which means that the

muscle of the right ventricle becomes thickened

Signs and symptoms:

- Some newborns with TOF may have no signs or symptoms, while others may have severe symptoms, such as:
- Rapid breathing or difficulty breathing
- Fatigue or poor feeding
- Persistent or recurrent lung infections
- Heart murmur
- Swelling of the legs, feet, or abdomen
- Bluish skin (cyanosis)

Diagnosis:

- The most common way to diagnose TOF is through an echocardiogram (a type of ultrasound that uses sound waves to create images of the heart) which can be done as early as the first days of life.
- Other diagnostic tools may include a chest x-ray, electrocardiogram (ECG), and a cardiac catheterization (a procedure that uses a thin tube to look inside the heart and blood vessels).

Treatment:

- Dependent on the size of the defect, the symptoms it causes, and the child's overall health.
- Smaller defects may not require treatment and may close on their own over time.
- Larger defects may require surgery to repair the hole, which can be done through open heart surgery or by a

catheter-based procedure.
- Some of the surgical options include :
  - a complete repair which is a procedure that corrects all four defects in the heart and can be done in the first months of life
  - a palliative procedure, which helps to alleviate the symptoms caused by the defects but does not correct them.

Prognosis:

- The prognosis depends on the size of the defect, the symptoms it causes and the overall health of the child.
- With proper treatment and management, most children with TOF can lead normal, healthy lives.
- After surgical correction, many children with TOF have a good long-term outlook, although some may experience complications such as arrhythmias or other heart problems.
- Children with TOF may require lifelong follow-up care with a pediatric cardiologist to monitor for any potential complications and to ensure that the repair is working as it should.

Tetralogy of Fallot is considered a complex heart defect and a multidisciplinary approach is usually taken to ensure the best outcome for the child, which can include a team of pediatric cardiologists, surgeons, anesthesiologists, nurses, and other specialists.

Coarctation of the Aorta (CoA)

Coarctation of the aorta (CoA) is a congenital heart defect that occurs when there is a narrowing of the aorta, the main blood vessel that carries oxygen-rich blood from the heart to the body. This narrowing can cause reduced blood flow to the body, particularly to the lower half of the body.

Signs and symptoms:

- Some newborns with CoA may have no signs or symptoms, while others may have severe symptoms, such as:
- Rapid breathing or difficulty breathing
- Fatigue or poor feeding
- Persistent or recurrent lung infections
- Heart murmur
- Swelling of the legs, feet, or abdomen
- Bluish skin (cyanosis)

Diagnosis:

- The most common way to diagnose CoA is through an echocardiogram (a type of ultrasound that uses sound waves to create images of the heart) which can be done as early as the first days of life.
- Other diagnostic tools may include a chest x-ray, electrocardiogram (ECG), and a cardiac catheterization (a procedure that uses a thin tube to look inside the heart and blood vessels).

Treatment:

- Treatment for CoA depends on the size of the defect, the symptoms it causes, and the child's overall health.

- Smaller defects may not require treatment and may close on their own over time.
- Larger defects may require surgery to repair the narrowing of the aorta, which can be done through open heart surgery or by a catheter-based procedure.
- Medications such as blood pressure medications and diuretics may be prescribed to manage symptoms and blood pressure and increase blood flow to the lower body

Prognosis:

- The prognosis for a newborn with CoA depends on the size of the defect, the symptoms it causes, and the overall health of the child.
- Smaller defects may not cause any symptoms and may close on their own over time, resulting in a good prognosis.
- Larger defects may cause symptoms such as hypertension, fatigue, and heart failure and may require surgery. The prognosis after surgery is generally good, but depends on the child's overall health and the specific circumstances of the surgery.

The prognosis for a newborn with CoA may change over time and that it's important for the parents and caregivers to consult with a pediatric cardiologist for regular check-ups and follow-up care. Children with CoA may require lifelong follow-up care with a pediatric cardiologist to monitor for any potential complications and to ensure that the repair is working as it should. It's also worth mentioning that Coarctation of the aorta is considered a complex heart defect and a multidisciplinary approach is usually taken to ensure the best outcome for the child, which can include a team of pediatric cardiologists, surgeons, anesthesiologists, nurses, and other specialists. It's also important to note that some children with CoA may also have other underlying heart defects that also need to be addressed.

Transposition of the Great Vessels (TGA)

Transposition of the great vessels (TGA) is a congenital heart defect that occurs when the aorta and pulmonary artery are switched in position. This means that the aorta, which should carry oxygen-rich blood from the heart to the body, is connected to the right ventricle, and the pulmonary artery, which should carry oxygen-poor blood from the heart to the lungs, is connected to the left ventricle. This results in a lack of oxygen-rich blood reaching the body.

Signs and symptoms:

- Some newborns with TGA may have no signs or symptoms, while others may have severe symptoms, such as:
- Rapid breathing or difficulty breathing
- Fatigue or poor feeding
- Persistent or recurrent lung infections
- Heart murmur
- Swelling of the legs, feet, or abdomen
- Bluish skin (cyanosis)

Diagnosis:

- The most common way to diagnose TGA is through an echocardiogram (a type of ultrasound that uses sound waves to create images of the heart) which can be done as early as the first days of life.
- Other diagnostic tools may include a chest x-ray, electrocardiogram (ECG), and a cardiac catheterization (a procedure that uses a thin tube to look inside the heart

and blood vessels).

Treatment:

- Treatment for TGA is usually surgery, which is done to correct the position of the great vessels and improve the blood flow.
- Surgery is usually done shortly after birth and is done by an experienced congenital heart surgeon.
- In some cases, a temporary surgical procedure such as a balloon atrial septostomy may be done before the definitive surgical procedure.

Prognosis:

- The prognosis for a newborn with TGA depends on the size of the defect, the symptoms it causes, and the overall health of the child.
- With proper treatment and management, most children with TGA can lead normal, healthy lives.
- After surgical correction, many children with TGA have a good long-term outlook, although some may experience complications such as arrhythmias or other heart problems.
- Children with TGA may require lifelong follow-up care with a pediatric cardiologist to monitor for any potential complications and to ensure that the repair is working as it should.

Transposition of the Great vessels is considered a complex heart defect and a multidisciplinary approach is usually taken to ensure the best outcome for the child, which can include a team of pediatric cardiologists, surgeons, anesthesiologists, nurses, and other specialists. Some children with TGA may also have other underlying heart defects that also need to be addressed. It's also important to note that the first hours and days after birth are crucial for newborns with TGA, and they may require special care in a neonatal intensive care unit (NICU) before and after surgery.

Hypoplastic Left Heart Syndrome (HLHS)

Hypoplastic left heart syndrome (HLHS) is a congenital heart defect that occurs when the left side of the heart is underdeveloped. This means that the left ventricle, the aorta, and the aortic valve are smaller than normal and unable to pump blood effectively. This results in a lack of oxygen-rich blood reaching the body.

Signs and symptoms:

- Some newborns with HLHS may have no signs or symptoms, while others may have severe symptoms, such as:
- Rapid breathing or difficulty breathing
- Fatigue or poor feeding
- Persistent or recurrent lung infections
- Heart murmur
- Swelling of the legs, feet, or abdomen
- Bluish skin (cyanosis)

Diagnosis:

- The most common way to diagnose HLHS is through an echocardiogram (a type of ultrasound that uses sound waves to create images of the heart) which can be done as early as the first days of life.

- Other diagnostic tools may include a chest x-ray, electrocardiogram (ECG), and a cardiac catheterization (a procedure that uses a thin tube to look inside the heart and blood vessels).

Treatment:

- HLHS treatment is usually a three-stage surgical procedure called the Norwood procedure, which is done to improve the blood flow.
- The first stage is done shortly after birth and involves connecting the right ventricle to the aorta to provide blood flow to the body.
- The second stage is usually done between 3-6 months of age and involves connecting the pulmonary artery to the aorta.
- The third stage is usually done between 18-24 months of age and involves reconstructing the aorta and creating a new valve.
- Medications such as blood pressure medications and diuretics may be prescribed to manage symptoms and blood pressure and increase blood flow to the body.

Prognosis:

- The prognosis for a newborn with HLHS depends on the size of the defect, the symptoms it causes, and the overall health of the child.
- With proper treatment and management, most children with HLHS can lead normal, healthy lives.
- After surgical correction, many children with HLHS have a good long-term outlook, although some may experience complications such as arrhythmias or other heart problems.

- Children with HLHS may require lifelong follow-up care with a pediatric cardiologist to monitor for any potential complications and to ensure that the repair is working as it should.

Hypoplastic Left Heart Syndrome is considered a complex heart defect and a multidisciplinary approach is usually taken to ensure the best outcome for the child, which can include a team of pediatric cardiologists, surgeons, anesthesiologists, nurses, and other specialists.

Pulmonary Stenosis (PS)

Pulmonary stenosis (PS) is a congenital heart defect that occurs when the pulmonary valve, which controls the flow of blood from the right ventricle to the lungs, is narrowed or obstructed. This can cause difficulty pumping blood to the lungs, leading to a lack of oxygen-rich blood reaching the body.

Signs and symptoms:

- Some newborns with PS may have no signs or symptoms, while others may have severe symptoms, such as:
- Rapid breathing or difficulty breathing
- Fatigue or poor feeding
- Persistent or recurrent lung infections
- Heart murmur
- Swelling of the legs, feet, or abdomen
- Bluish skin (cyanosis)

Diagnosis:

- PS is most commonly diagnosed with echocardiogram (a type of ultrasound that uses sound waves to create images of the heart) which can be done as early as the first days of life.

- Other diagnostic tools may include a chest x-ray, electrocardiogram (ECG), and a cardiac catheterization (a procedure that uses a thin tube to look inside the heart and blood vessels).

Treatment:

- Treatment for PS depends on the severity of the obstruction and the symptoms it causes.
- In mild cases, no treatment may be needed, and the baby may be monitored regularly by a pediatric cardiologist.
- In moderate to severe cases, treatment may include surgery to repair or replace the pulmonary valve, which can be done through open-heart surgery or by a catheter-based procedure.
- Medications such as blood pressure medications may be prescribed to manage symptoms and blood pressure.

Prognosis:

- Prognosis for a newborn with PS depends on the severity of the obstruction, the symptoms it causes, and the overall health of the child.
- With proper treatment and management, most children with PS can lead normal, healthy lives.
- After surgical correction, many children with PS have a good long-term outlook, although some may experience complications such as arrhythmias or other heart problems.
- Children with PS may require lifelong follow-up care with a pediatric cardiologist to monitor for any potential complications and to ensure that the repair is working as it should.

Pulmonary Stenosis is considered a complex heart defect and a multidisciplinary approach is usually taken to ensure the best outcome for the child, which can include a team of pediatric cardiologists, surgeons, anesthesiologists, nurses, and other specialists.

Aortic Stenosis (AS)

Aortic stenosis (AS) is a congenital heart defect that occurs when the aortic valve, which controls the flow of blood from the left ventricle to the body, is narrowed or obstructed. This can cause difficulty pumping blood to the body, leading to a lack of oxygen-rich blood reaching the body.

Signs and symptoms:

- Some newborns with AS may have no signs or symptoms, while others may have severe symptoms, such as:
- Rapid breathing or difficulty breathing
- Fatigue or poor feeding
- Persistent or recurrent lung infections
- Heart murmur
- Swelling of the legs, feet, or abdomen
- Bluish skin (cyanosis)

Diagnosis:

- The most common way to diagnose AS is through an echocardiogram (a type of ultrasound that uses sound waves to create images of the heart) which can be done as early as the first days of life.
- Other diagnostic tools may include a chest x-ray, electrocardiogram (ECG), and a cardiac catheterization (a procedure that uses a thin tube to look inside the heart and blood vessels).

Treatment:

- Treatment for AS depends on the severity of the obstruction and the symptoms it causes.
- In mild cases, no treatment may be needed, and the baby may be monitored regularly by a pediatric cardiologist.
- In moderate to severe cases, treatment may include surgery to repair or replace the aortic valve, which can be done through open-heart surgery or by a catheter-based procedure.
- Medications such as blood pressure medications may be prescribed to manage symptoms and blood pressure.Prognosis:
- The prognosis for a newborn with AS depends on the severity of the obstruction, the symptoms it causes, and the overall health of the child.
- With proper treatment and management, most children with AS can lead normal, healthy lives.
- After surgical correction, many children with AS have a good long-term outlook, although some may experience complications such as arrhythmias or other heart problems.
- Children with AS may require lifelong follow-up care with a pediatric cardiologist to monitor for any potential complications and to ensure that the repair is working as it should.

Aortic Stenosis is considered a complex heart defect and a multidisciplinary approach is usually taken to ensure the best outcome for the child, which can include a team of pediatric cardiologists, surgeons, anesthesiologists, nurses, and other specialists.

Congenital Heart Block (CHB)

Congenital heart block (CHB) is a rare congenital birth defect that affects the electrical system of the heart. It occurs when the electrical signals that control the heart's rhythm do not pass properly from the mother's heart to the fetus's heart. This can cause the fetus's heart to beat too slowly, which can lead to heart failure and other serious complications.

Diagnosis: CHB is typically diagnosed during prenatal ultrasound, by a physical examination of the fetus's heart rate and rhythm. It can also be diagnosed after birth, by a physical examination of the newborn's heart rate and rhythm.

Signs and Symptoms:

- Slow heart rate (bradycardia)
- Heart failure
- Blue color to the skin, nails, and lips (cyanosis)
- Fatigue
- Shortness of breath
- Poor feeding

Treatment:

- Treatment for CHB typically involves the use of a pacemaker, which is a small device that sends electrical signals to the heart to help it beat at a normal rate.
- The pacemaker is typically implanted shortly after birth.
- Other treatments that may be necessary include medications to help the heart pump more effectively and/ or oxygen therapy.
- In some cases, surgery may be necessary to repair or replace the heart's electrical system.

Prognosis:

- The prognosis for CHB depends on the severity of the condition, the success of the pacemaker treatment, and the presence of any other heart defects.
- With proper treatment, most children with CHB can achieve normal heart function and a good quality of life.
- However, there is a risk of complications such as infection, bleeding, or damage to the heart's electrical system.
- Children with CHB may require lifelong follow-up care with a team of healthcare professionals including pediatric cardiologists, electrophysiologists and pediatricians to monitor for any potential complications and to ensure that the pacemaker is working properly.

Congenital heart block is a serious condition that requires prompt diagnosis and treatment, as it can lead to permanent damage to the heart's electrical system and heart failure if left untreated. With proper treatment, most children with CHB can achieve normal heart function and a good quality of life, but they may require lifelong follow-up care to monitor for any potential complications and to ensure that the pacemaker is working properly.

Arrhythmias

Arrhythmias are abnormal heart rhythms that occur in children. They can range from mild, asymptomatic cases to life-threatening arrhythmias that require immediate medical attention.

Diagnosis: Arrhythmias are diagnosed through a combination of medical history, physical examination, and diagnostic tests, including electrocardiogram (ECG) and echocardiogram.

Signs and Symptoms: The signs and symptoms of arrhythmias can vary widely, depending on the type and severity of the arrhythmia. Some common signs and symptoms include:

- Rapid heartbeat
- Slow heartbeat
- Palpitations (sensations of skipped or extra heart beats)
- Chest pain
- Shortness of breath
- Fatigue
- Fainting or near-fainting

Prognosis: The prognosis of arrhythmias in the pediatric population depends on the underlying cause, type, and severity of the arrhythmia. Some arrhythmias are benign and require no treatment, while others may require medication, surgery, or other interventions to manage symptoms and prevent complications. With proper management and treatment, most children with arrhythmias can lead normal, healthy lives.

Treatment: The treatment of arrhythmias depends on the type and severity of the arrhythmia, as well as the age and overall health of the child. Treatment options may include:

- Medications to regulate heart rate and rhythm
- Catheter ablation, a minimally invasive procedure that uses radiofrequency energy to destroy the heart tissue responsible for the arrhythmia
- Pacemaker implantation, which can help regulate the heart rate and rhythm in children with slow heart rates
- Surgery, such as the Maze procedure, which is used to treat atrial fibrillation in some cases

In addition to these medical interventions, lifestyle modifications, such as avoiding caffeine and other stimulants, getting regular exercise, and managing stress, can also help manage pediatric arrhythmias. Close monitoring and follow-up with a pediatric cardiologist are important for ensuring the ongoing health and well-being of children with arrhythmias.

Cardiomyopathy

Pediatric cardiomyopathy is a condition in which the heart muscle becomes enlarged, thickened, or stiff, which can lead to reduced heart function and heart failure. The condition can be caused by a variety of factors, including genetics, viral infections, and metabolic disorders.

Diagnosis: Cardiomyopathy is diagnosed through a combination of medical history, physical examination, and diagnostic tests, including echocardiogram, electrocardiogram (ECG), and cardiac MRI. Genetic testing may also be recommended in some cases.

Signs and Symptoms: The signs and symptoms of cardiomyopathy can vary widely, depending on the type and severity of the condition. Some common signs and symptoms include:

- Rapid heartbeat
- Slow heartbeat
- Shortness of breath
- Fatigue
- Chest pain
- Swelling in the legs, feet, or abdomen
- Fainting or near-fainting

Prognosis: The prognosis of cardiomyopathy depends on the underlying cause, type, and severity of the condition. With proper management and treatment, many children with cardiomyopathy can live relatively normal lives. However, severe cases may require heart transplantation or other advanced treatments.

Treatment: The treatment of cardiomyopathy depends on the type and severity of the condition, as well as the age and overall health of the child. Treatment options may include:

- Medications to improve heart function, regulate heart rhythm, or reduce symptoms
- Lifestyle modifications, such as limiting physical activity and avoiding certain medications
- Surgical interventions, such as septal myectomy or ventricular assist devices
- Heart transplantation, in severe cases

In addition to medical interventions, children with cardiomyopathy require close monitoring and follow-up with a pediatric cardiologist, as well as ongoing management of any underlying conditions that may be contributing to the condition. Familial screening and genetic counseling may also be recommended in some cases to identify and manage any potential genetic risks for cardiomyopathy in family members.

Rheumatic Fever

Rheumatic fever is an inflammatory disease that can develop after a streptococcal (strep) infection, such as strep throat or scarlet fever. It is caused by an immune response to the strep infection, which can attack the heart, joints, skin, and brain. The exact cause of rheumatic fever is not fully understood, but it is thought to be triggered by a combination of genetic and environmental factors.

The signs and symptoms of pediatric rheumatic fever can vary depending on the affected organs, but they can include:

- Joint pain and swelling
- Fever
- Fatigue

- Skin rash
- Chest pain
- Shortness of breath
- Heart murmur
- Abnormal heart rhythm

To diagnose rheumatic fever, a pediatrician will typically perform a physical examination and ask about the child's symptoms. The diagnosis can be confirmed by blood tests (ASO, Anti-DNAase B, Anti-Streptolysin O) and Echocardiogram.

The treatment for rheumatic fever typically includes:

- Antibiotics to treat the underlying strep infection
- Anti-inflammatory medications to reduce inflammation and swelling in the joints
- Medications to control heart symptoms, such as beta-blockers or ACE inhibitors
- Physical therapy to help with joint pain and stiffness
- Surgery in some cases
- Long-term preventive therapy with antibiotics to prevent recurrences

Prognosis for rheumatic fever can vary depending on the severity of the disease, how quickly the child is diagnosed and treated, and whether any complications occur. With proper treatment and care, most children will make a full recovery and prevent future recurrences. However, in some cases, rheumatic fever can lead to serious complications such as heart damage, joint damage, and brain damage. It's important to seek medical attention if a child is showing any signs or symptoms of rheumatic fever and to keep up-to-date with vaccinations to prevent the disease.

Kawasaki Disease

Kawasaki disease is a rare but serious childhood illness that causes inflammation in the blood vessels throughout the body. The exact cause of Kawasaki disease is not known, but it is thought to be an autoimmune disorder triggered by an infection. The disease affects mostly children under 5 years old and it is more common in boys than girls.

The signs and symptoms of Kawasaki disease can vary, but they typically include:

- High fever that lasts for at least 5 days
- Rash
- Swollen hands and feet
- Swollen lymph nodes in the neck
- Redness and swelling of the whites of the eyes
- Cracked, dry lips and redness of the tongue
- Irritability
- Joint pain
- Swelling of the coronary artery (in severe cases)

To diagnose Kawasaki disease, a pediatrician will typically perform a physical examination and ask about the child's symptoms. The diagnosis can be confirmed by blood tests (Elevated ESR, CRP, Platelet count) and Echocardiogram.

The treatment for Kawasaki disease typically includes:

- High-dose of aspirin to reduce inflammation and swelling in the blood vessels
- Intravenous immunoglobulin (IVIG) to reduce inflammation in the blood vessels
- Medications to control fever
- Close monitoring for any signs of heart problems

Prognosis for Kawasaki disease can vary depending on the severity of the disease, how quickly the child is diagnosed and treated, and whether any complications occur. With proper treatment and care, most children will make a full recovery and prevent future recurrences. However, in some cases, Kawasaki disease can lead to serious complications such as heart damage, joint damage, and brain damage.

Pulmonary Hypertension

Pediatric pulmonary hypertension (PH) is a condition in which there is increased pressure in the pulmonary arteries, which carry blood from the heart to the lungs. This can lead to heart failure and other serious complications if left untreated.

Diagnosis: Pulmonary Hypertension is diagnosed through a combination of medical history, physical examination, and diagnostic tests, including echocardiogram, electrocardiogram (ECG), chest X-ray, and right heart catheterization.

Signs and Symptoms: The signs and symptoms of pulnonary hypertension can vary widely, depending on the type and severity of the condition. Some common signs and symptoms include:

- Shortness of breath
- Fatigue
- Chest pain
- Fainting or near-fainting
- Bluish lips, fingers, or toes (cyanosis)
- Swelling in the legs, feet, or abdomen
- Rapid heartbeat

Prognosis: The prognosis of pulmonary hypertention depends

on the underlying cause, type, and severity of the condition. Early diagnosis and treatment can improve outcomes, but severe cases can lead to heart failure and other serious complications. With proper management and treatment, many children with PH can lead normal, healthy lives.

Treatment: The treatment of pulmonary hypertension depends on the underlying cause, type, and severity of the condition, as well as the age and overall health of the child. Treatment options may include:

- Medications to dilate blood vessels, reduce blood pressure, or improve heart function
- Oxygen therapy, to improve breathing and increase oxygen levels in the blood
- Surgery, such as pulmonary thromboendarterectomy or atrial septostomy
- Lung transplant, in severe cases

In addition to medical interventions, children with pulmonary hypertension require close monitoring and follow-up with a pediatric cardiologist, as well as ongoing management of any underlying conditions that may be contributing to the condition. Lifestyle modifications, such as avoiding strenuous physical activity and maintaining a healthy weight, may also be recommended.

Syncope

Syncope (fainting) secondary to a cardiac cause is a condition in which a child loses consciousness due to a sudden decrease in blood flow to the brain as a result of a cardiac problem. This can be caused by a variety of conditions, including arrhythmias, heart block, structural heart defects, or other cardiac abnormalities.

Diagnosis: Diagnosis of syncope secondary to a cardiac cause involves a thorough medical history, physical examination, and diagnostic tests, including electrocardiogram (ECG), echocardiogram, and Holter monitoring (a portable ECG device worn for 24-48 hours to monitor heart rhythm). Other tests such as exercise stress testing, tilt table testing, and cardiac MRI may also be ordered by the pediatric cardiologist.

Signs and Symptoms: The signs and symptoms of syncope secondary to a cardiac cause can include:

- Sudden loss of consciousness
- Paleness or cyanosis (bluish discoloration of the skin)
- Rapid or irregular heartbeat
- Chest pain or discomfort
- Shortness of breath
- Dizziness or lightheadedness

Prognosis: The prognosis of syncope secondary to a cardiac cause depends on the underlying condition causing the syncope. Some conditions may be treated effectively with medication or surgery, while others may require more aggressive interventions, such as cardiac ablation or implantation of a pacemaker or defibrillator. In some cases, the condition may be life-threatening and require immediate emergency treatment.

Treatment: Treatment of syncope secondary to a cardiac cause depends on the underlying condition causing the syncope. Treatment options may include:

- Medications to regulate heart rhythm, improve heart function, or reduce symptoms
- Surgery, such as cardiac ablation or implantation of a pacemaker or defibrillator
- Lifestyle modifications, such as avoiding certain triggers (such as dehydration or prolonged standing) that can lead to syncope

In addition to medical interventions, children with syncope secondary to a cardiac cause require close monitoring and follow-up with a pediatric cardiologist, as well as ongoing management of any underlying conditions that may be contributing to the syncope.

Chest Pain

Most commonly, chest pain in the pediatric population is generally related to musculoskeletal cause and mostly benign, however, it can be caused by a variety of conditions, including arrhythmias, myocarditis, pericarditis, coronary artery anomalies, or other structural heart defects.

Diagnosis: Diagnosis of chest pain secondary to a cardiac cause involves a thorough medical history, physical examination, and diagnostic tests, including electrocardiogram (ECG), echocardiogram, chest X-ray, and cardiac MRI or CT scan. Blood tests and stress testing may also be ordered by the pediatric cardiologist.

Signs and Symptoms: The signs and symptoms of chest pain secondary to a cardiac cause can include:

- Pain or discomfort in the chest, which may feel like pressure, squeezing, or burning
- Pain or discomfort that spreads to the neck, jaw, arms, back, or shoulders
- Shortness of breath
- Rapid or irregular heartbeat
- Dizziness or lightheadedness
- Fainting or near-fainting
- Bluish lips or fingers (cyanosis)

Prognosis: The prognosis of chest pain secondary to a

cardiac cause depends on the underlying condition causing the chest pain. Some conditions may be treated effectively with medication or lifestyle modifications, while others may require more aggressive interventions, such as surgery or catheterization. In some cases, the condition may be life-threatening and require immediate emergency treatment.

Treatment: Treatment of chest pain secondary to a cardiac cause depends on the underlying condition causing the chest pain. Treatment options may include:

- Medications to regulate heart rhythm, improve heart function, or reduce symptoms
- Surgery, such as coronary artery bypass grafting or valve replacement
- Catheterization, such as balloon angioplasty or stent placement
- Lifestyle modifications, such as maintaining a healthy weight, avoiding tobacco and alcohol, and managing stress

In addition to medical interventions, children with chest pain secondary to a cardiac cause require close monitoring and follow-up with a pediatric cardiologist, as well as ongoing management of any underlying conditions that may be contributing to the chest pain.

Hypertension

Hypertension, or high blood pressure, is a condition in which the force of blood against the walls of the arteries is too high. It is diagnosed based on repeated elevated blood pressure readings on at least three separate occasions.

Diagnosis: The diagnosis of hypertension is typically made through measuring the child's blood pressure and comparing it to age, sex, and height-specific norms. In addition to in-office blood pressure readings, ambulatory blood pressure monitoring and home blood pressure monitoring may be used to confirm the diagnosis.

Signs and Symptoms: In many cases, hypertension has no signs or symptoms and is only detected through routine blood pressure screening. However, some children with hypertension may experience symptoms such as headaches, dizziness, blurry vision, chest pain, shortness of breath, and nosebleeds.

Prognosis: The prognosis of hypertension depends on the underlying cause and the severity of the condition. If left untreated, hypertension can lead to damage to the heart, kidneys, blood vessels, and other organs. However, with proper management and treatment, most children with hypertension can lead normal, healthy lives.

Treatment: Treatment of hypertension involves a combination of lifestyle modifications and medication. Lifestyle modifications include maintaining a healthy weight, eating a healthy diet, getting regular physical activity, reducing salt and caffeine intake, and managing stress. Medications may be prescribed to help lower blood pressure and manage any underlying conditions that may be contributing to hypertension.

Prognosis: The prognosis of hypertension depends on the underlying cause and the severity of the condition. If left untreated, hypertension can lead to damage to the heart, kidneys, blood vessels, and other organs. However, with proper management and treatment, most children with hypertension can lead normal, healthy lives.

Overall, the diagnosis and management of pediatric hypertension should be managed by a pediatrician or pediatric cardiologist to ensure proper evaluation, treatment, and monitoring of the child's condition.

Lipid Disorders

Lipid disorders affecting the heart refers to abnormal levels of lipids, or fats, in the blood that can lead to the development of cardiovascular disease. The most common lipid disorder in children is familial hypercholesterolemia, which is a genetic condition that causes high levels of LDL (low-density lipoprotein) cholesterol.

Diagnosis: The diagnosis of a lipid disorder is made through a blood test that measures cholesterol and other lipid levels. A family history of high cholesterol or heart disease may also be considered.
Signs and Symptoms:

Pediatric lipid disorders affecting the heart usually do not have any symptoms. However, high levels of LDL cholesterol over time can lead to the development of atherosclerosis, or plaque buildup in the arteries. Atherosclerosis can lead to heart disease, heart attack, or stroke.

Prognosis: The prognosis of lipid disorders affecting the heart depends on the underlying cause and the severity of the condition. If left untreated, these conditions can lead to serious cardiovascular disease. However, with proper management and treatment, many children with lipid disorders can prevent or delay the onset of cardiovascular disease.

Treatment: Treatment of lipid disorders affecting the heart typically involves a combination of lifestyle modifications and medication. Lifestyle modifications may include maintaining a healthy weight, eating a healthy diet, getting regular physical activity, and avoiding tobacco use. Medications may be prescribed to help lower cholesterol levels and prevent the development of cardiovascular disease.

Prognosis: The prognosis of lipid disorders affecting the heart depends on the underlying cause and the severity of the condition. If left untreated, these conditions can lead to serious cardiovascular disease. However, with proper management and treatment, many children with lipid disorders can prevent or delay the onset of cardiovascular disease.

CHAPTER 2

Gastroenterology

Pediatric gastroenterology is a medical specialty that deals with the diagnosis and treatment of digestive system disorders in children. Some of the common diagnoses that are treated by pediatric gastroenterologists include:

1. Gastroesophageal reflux disease (GERD): This is a condition in which stomach acid backs up into the esophagus, causing heartburn, nausea, and other symptoms.
2. Inflammatory bowel disease (IBD): This is a chronic condition that causes inflammation and damage to the digestive tract, including Crohn's disease and ulcerative colitis.
3. Celiac disease: This is an autoimmune disorder that causes damage to the small intestine when gluten is ingested, leading to malabsorption of nutrients.
4. Functional gastrointestinal disorders: These are disorders in which the digestive tract appears to be normal, but the child experiences symptoms such as abdominal pain, constipation, or diarrhea.
5. Liver disease: This includes a variety of conditions such as hepatitis, cirrhosis, and liver failure.
6. Pancreatic disease: This includes conditions such as pancreatitis, cystic fibrosis, and other disorders that

affect the pancreas.

7.   Gastrointestinal infections: These are infections that affect the digestive system, such as gastroenteritis or food poisoning.

8.   Motility disorders: These are disorders that affect the movement of food through the digestive system, such as gastroparesis or intestinal dysmotility.

9.   Intestinal polyps: These are growths on the lining of the intestine that can be benign or cancerous.

10. Malabsorption syndromes: These are disorders in which the body is unable to absorb certain nutrients, such as lactose intolerance or short bowel syndrome.

Gastroesophageal Reflux Disease (GERD)

Gastroesophageal reflux disease (GERD) in children is a condition in which stomach acid flows back up into the esophagus, causing discomfort and other symptoms. Here is a brief overview of the diagnosis, signs, symptoms, treatment, and prognosis of pediatric GERD:

Diagnosis: GERD is typically diagnosed based on a combination of clinical history, symptoms, and physical examination. In some cases, additional testing may be required, such as a pH monitoring test or an upper gastrointestinal endoscopy.

Signs and symptoms:

The signs and symptoms of GERD can vary, but typically include:

- Frequent vomiting
- Refusing to eat or difficulty eating
- Irritability or fussiness during or after feedings
- Poor weight gain or failure to thrive

- Abdominal pain or discomfort
- Chronic cough or wheezing
- Hoarseness or sore throat
- Tooth erosion
- Bad breath

Treatment: Treatment for GERD typically involves a combination of lifestyle changes, medication, and sometimes surgery. Some of the most common treatment options include:

- Feeding changes, such as smaller, more frequent feedings or thicker formula
- Medications to reduce stomach acid, such as proton pump inhibitors (PPIs) or H2 blockers
- Medications to improve gastric emptying, such as prokinetic agents
- Surgery, such as a fundoplication, if lifestyle changes and medications are not effective

Prognosis: The prognosis for GERD is generally good, with most children experiencing improvement in symptoms with treatment. However, some children may require ongoing treatment or monitoring, and some may experience complications, such as esophagitis, strictures, or respiratory problems.

It is important to note that GERD can also be a sign of other underlying conditions, such as a hiatal hernia, eosinophilic esophagitis, or gastrointestinal motility disorders.

Inflammatory Bowel Disease (IBD)

Pediatric inflammatory bowel disease (IBD) is a chronic inflammatory condition that affects the digestive tract of children. Here is a brief overview of the diagnosis, signs, symptoms, treatment, and prognosis of pediatric IBD:

Diagnosis: IBD is typically diagnosed based on a combination of clinical history, symptoms, and diagnostic tests. Diagnostic tests may include blood tests, stool tests, endoscopy, and imaging studies such as X-rays or magnetic resonance enterography.

Signs and symptoms: The signs and symptoms of IBD can vary depending on the type of IBD (Crohn's disease or ulcerative colitis), the location and extent of inflammation, and the severity of the disease. Some of the most common signs and symptoms of pediatric IBD include:

- Diarrhea (sometimes with blood)
- Abdominal pain and cramping
- Weight loss and poor growth
- Loss of appetite
- Fatigue and weakness
- Anemia
- Delayed puberty or stunted growth
- Joint pain or swelling
- Skin rash
- Eye inflammation

Treatment: The treatment of IBD typically involves a combination of medication and dietary modifications. Some of the most common medications used to treat pediatric IBD include:

- Aminosalicylates (e.g. mesalamine)
- Corticosteroids (e.g. prednisone)
- Immunosuppressants (e.g. azathioprine, 6-mercaptopurine)
- Biologic therapies (e.g. infliximab, adalimumab)
- Antibiotics
- Anti-diarrheal medications

Dietary modifications may include avoiding certain foods, increasing fiber intake, and using specialized formulas or nutritional supplements.

In some cases, surgery may be necessary to treat complications of IBD or to remove affected portions of the bowel.

Prognosis: The prognosis for IBD varies depending on the type and severity of the disease, as well as the individual child's response to treatment. With proper treatment, many children with IBD are able to achieve remission and live relatively normal lives. However, some children may require ongoing treatment and monitoring, and may experience complications such as growth delay, malnutrition, or increased risk of certain cancers.

Celiac Disease

Celiac disease is an autoimmune disorder that affects the digestive system. It is caused by an immune response to gluten, a protein found in wheat, barley, and rye. When a person with celiac disease consumes gluten, their immune system attacks the small intestine, causing damage to the villi (small finger-like projections) that line the intestine. This damage makes it difficult for the body to absorb nutrients from food.

The signs and symptoms of celiac disease can vary depending on the child's age, but they typically include:

- Diarrhea
- Constipation
- Abdominal pain
- Bloating
- Gas
- Weight loss
- Fatigue
- Anemia
- Delayed growth and development

- Skin rash (dermatitis herpetiformis)

To diagnose celiac disease, a pediatrician will typically perform a physical examination and ask about the child's symptoms. Additional tests such as blood tests (tTG-IgA, EMA-IgA, DGP-IgA) and biopsy of the small intestine can also be done to confirm the diagnosis

The treatment for celiac disease is a gluten-free diet. This means removing all sources of gluten from the diet, including wheat, barley, and rye. This can be difficult, but with the help of a dietitian, it's possible to provide a balanced and nutritious diet.

Prognosis for celiac disease can vary depending on how quickly the child is diagnosed and treated, and whether any complications occur. With proper treatment and care, most children with celiac disease will be able to lead normal lives, but it is important to follow a strict gluten-free diet for life, otherwise, it can lead to serious complications such as malnutrition, osteoporosis, and other autoimmune disorders.

Functional Gastrointestinal Disorders (FGIDs)

Functional gastrointestinal disorders (FGIDs) are a group of conditions that affect the digestive system and cause chronic or recurrent symptoms without evidence of structural or biochemical abnormalities. These conditions are often referred to as functional disorders or functional dyspepsia. Here is a brief overview of the diagnosis, signs, symptoms, treatment, and prognosis of pediatric functional dysfunction disorders:

Diagnosis: The diagnosis of FGIDs is typically made based on clinical history, symptoms, and exclusion of other possible causes. Diagnostic tests may be ordered to rule out other conditions, but there is no specific test or biomarker for FGIDs. Signs and symptoms:

The signs and symptoms of FGIDs can vary depending on the specific disorder, but may include:

- Abdominal pain or discomfort
- Bloating or distention
- Nausea or vomiting
- Changes in bowel habits (constipation, diarrhea, or alternating)
- Loss of appetite
- Early satiety (feeling full after eating a small amount)
- Heartburn or acid reflux
- Difficulty swallowing

Treatment: The treatment of FGIDs typically involves a combination of lifestyle modifications, dietary changes, and medication. Some of the most common treatment options include:

- Dietary modifications (e.g. avoiding trigger foods, increasing fiber intake)
- Stress management techniques (e.g. mindfulness, relaxation exercises)
- Medications to relieve symptoms (e.g. antacids, prokinetics, laxatives)
- Cognitive behavioral therapy (CBT)
- Hypnotherapy

Prognosis: The prognosis for FGIDs varies depending on the severity of symptoms and the individual child's response to treatment. In many cases, symptoms can be managed effectively with lifestyle modifications and medication. However, some children may experience persistent symptoms that require ongoing treatment or management. The long-term outlook for pediatric FGIDs is generally good, and most children are able to lead normal lives with appropriate treatment and support.

Liver Disease

Pediatric liver disease refers to any condition that affects the liver in infants, children, or adolescents. The liver is an essential organ that performs various vital functions, such as producing bile, breaking down toxins and medications, and storing glucose. Pediatric liver diseases are relatively rare, but they can have severe consequences if left untreated. In this answer, we will discuss the common types, symptoms, diagnosis, and treatment of pediatric liver diseases.

Types of Pediatric Liver Disease:

1. Biliary Atresia: It is a rare congenital disease in which the bile ducts that carry bile from the liver to the intestine become blocked or damaged. This leads to a buildup of bile in the liver, causing inflammation and scarring. If left untreated, it can result in liver failure. Symptoms include yellowing of the skin and eyes (jaundice), dark urine, and pale stools.

2. Alagille Syndrome: It is a genetic disorder that affects multiple organs, including the liver. The condition causes the bile ducts to be narrower than usual, leading to a buildup of bile in the liver. This can cause liver damage, cirrhosis, and liver failure. Symptoms include jaundice, pale stools, and poor growth.

3. Alpha-1 Antitrypsin Deficiency: It is an inherited disorder that affects the production of alpha-1 antitrypsin, a protein that protects the liver from damage. In this condition, the liver produces a defective form of the protein, which can lead to liver damage, cirrhosis, and liver failure. Symptoms include jaundice, abdominal swelling, and poor growth.

4. Hepatitis: It is an inflammation of the liver caused by viral infections, autoimmune diseases, or exposure to

toxins. Symptoms include jaundice, fatigue, abdominal pain, and nausea.

5.   Wilson's Disease: It is a genetic disorder that affects the liver's ability to eliminate excess copper from the body. This leads to the buildup of copper in the liver, causing liver damage, cirrhosis, and liver failure. Symptoms include fatigue, abdominal pain, and tremors.

Symptoms: The symptoms of liver disease vary depending on the type and severity of the condition. Some of the common symptoms are:

- Jaundice
- Pale stools
- Dark urine
- Abdominal swelling or pain
- Nausea or vomiting
- Fatigue or weakness
- Poor appetite or weight loss
- Itchy skin
- Enlarged liver or spleen
- Bleeding or bruising easily
- Growth failure

Diagnosis: Pediatric liver diseases are diagnosed based on a combination of medical history, physical examination, and diagnostic tests. The doctor may perform blood tests to check for liver function, viral infections, or genetic disorders. Imaging tests like ultrasound, MRI, or CT scan may also be done to check for structural abnormalities in the liver. A liver biopsy may be required in some cases to examine the liver tissue for damage or inflammation.

Treatment: The treatment of pediatric liver disease depends on the type and severity of the condition. Some common treatments are:

1.   Medications: Certain medications may be prescribed

to treat the underlying condition or symptoms of liver disease. For example, antiviral medications are used to treat hepatitis, while steroids may be prescribed for autoimmune liver disease.

2.   Surgery: In some cases, surgery may be necessary to remove a damaged part of the liver or to perform a liver transplant.

3.   Nutritional Support: Children with liver disease may have poor growth and malnutrition due to poor nutrient absorption. Nutritional support, including specialized diets or supplements, may be required to maintain adequate nutrition.

4.   Management of Complications: Children with liver disease may develop complications like bleeding disorders or infections. Treatment may be required to

Pancreatic Disease

Pediatric pancreatic disease refers to any condition that affects the pancreas in infants, children, or adolescents. The pancreas is an important organ that produces digestive enzymes and hormones like insulin and glucagon. Pediatric pancreatic diseases are relatively rare but can have severe consequences if left untreated. In this answer, we will discuss the common types, symptoms, diagnosis, and treatment of pediatric pancreatic diseases.

Types of Pediatric Pancreatic Disease:

1.   Acute Pancreatitis: It is a sudden inflammation of the pancreas, which can be caused by various factors like infections, medications, or trauma. Symptoms include severe abdominal pain, nausea, vomiting, and fever.

2.   Chronic Pancreatitis: It is a long-term inflammation of the pancreas, which can be caused by alcohol abuse, autoimmune diseases, or genetic disorders. Symptoms include recurrent abdominal pain, diarrhea, weight loss,

and malnutrition.

3. Pancreatic Cysts: It is a fluid-filled sac that develops within the pancreas. Cysts can be benign or malignant and can cause symptoms like abdominal pain, nausea, vomiting, or jaundice.

4. Pancreatic Cancer: It is a rare but serious type of cancer that develops in the pancreas. Symptoms include abdominal pain, jaundice, weight loss, and fatigue.

Symptoms: The symptoms of pediatric pancreatic disease vary depending on the type and severity of the condition. Some common symptoms are:

- Abdominal pain or discomfort
- Nausea or vomiting
- Diarrhea or constipation
- Weight loss or poor growth
- Jaundice
- Fatigue or weakness
- Malnutrition
- Diabetes
- Fevers

Diagnosis: Pancreatic diseases are diagnosed based on a combination of medical history, physical examination, and diagnostic tests. The doctor may perform blood tests to check for pancreatic function, viral infections, or genetic disorders. Imaging tests like ultrasound, MRI, or CT scan may also be done to check for structural abnormalities in the pancreas. An endoscopic procedure may be required in some cases to examine the pancreas or to collect tissue samples for further analysis.

Treatment: The treatment of pancreatic disease depends on the type and severity of the condition. Some common treatments are:

1. Medications: Certain medications may be prescribed to

treat the underlying condition or symptoms of pancreatic disease. For example, pain relievers, antibiotics, or enzyme supplements may be prescribed to manage the symptoms of pancreatitis.

2. Surgery: In some cases, surgery may be necessary to remove a damaged part of the pancreas or to treat complications like pancreatic cysts or cancer.

3. Nutritional Support: Children with pancreatic disease may have poor growth and malnutrition due to poor nutrient absorption. Nutritional support, including specialized diets or supplements, may be required to maintain adequate nutrition.

4. Management of Complications: Children with pancreatic disease may develop complications like diabetes or infections. Treatment may be required to manage these complications and prevent further damage.

In conclusion, pancreatic disease is a relatively rare but serious condition that requires prompt diagnosis and treatment to prevent further damage.

Gastrointestinal Infections

Pediatric gastrointestinal infections refer to infections of the digestive system that affect infants, children, and adolescents. These infections can be caused by viruses, bacteria, parasites, or fungi and can cause a range of symptoms from mild to severe. In this answer, we will discuss the common types, symptoms, diagnosis, and treatment of pediatric gastrointestinal infections.

Types of Pediatric Gastrointestinal Infections:

1. Rotavirus Infection: Rotavirus is a common cause of gastroenteritis in infants and young children. Symptoms include vomiting, diarrhea, and fever.

2. Norovirus Infection: Norovirus is a highly contagious

virus that can cause outbreaks of gastroenteritis in schools, daycare centers, and other group settings. Symptoms include vomiting, diarrhea, and stomach cramps.

3.   Salmonella Infection: Salmonella is a type of bacteria that can cause food poisoning. Children can contract it by eating contaminated food or coming into contact with contaminated animals or their environment. Symptoms include diarrhea, fever, and abdominal cramps.

4.   Campylobacter Infection: Campylobacter is another type of bacteria that can cause food poisoning. Children can contract it by eating contaminated food or coming into contact with contaminated animals or their environment. Symptoms include diarrhea, fever, and abdominal cramps.

5.   Giardia Infection: Giardia is a parasite that can cause diarrhea, abdominal cramps, and weight loss in children who drink contaminated water.

Symptoms: The symptoms of pediatric gastrointestinal infections vary depending on the type and severity of the infection. Some common symptoms are:

- Abdominal pain or cramps
- Nausea or vomiting
- Diarrhea or constipation
- Fever
- Loss of appetite
- Dehydration
- Fatigue or weakness

Diagnosis: Pediatric gastrointestinal infections are diagnosed based on a combination of medical history, physical examination, and diagnostic tests. The doctor may perform stool tests to check for the presence of viruses, bacteria, parasites, or fungi. Blood tests may also be done to check for signs of infection or dehydration. Imaging tests like ultrasound, CT scan, or MRI may be required in some cases to check for structural abnormalities in the digestive system.

Treatment: The treatment of gastrointestinal infections depends on the type and severity of the infection. Some common treatments are:

1.   Fluid Replacement: Children with gastrointestinal infections may become dehydrated due to vomiting and diarrhea. Treatment may include oral or intravenous fluids to maintain hydration.
2.   Medications: Certain medications may be prescribed to treat the underlying infection or symptoms of gastrointestinal infections. For example, antibiotics may be prescribed to treat bacterial infections, and antiemetics may be prescribed to manage vomiting.
3.   Nutritional Support: Children with gastrointestinal infections may have poor appetite and malnutrition due to poor nutrient absorption. Nutritional support, including specialized diets or supplements, may be required to maintain adequate nutrition.
4.   Prevention: The best way to prevent pediatric gastrointestinal infections is to practice good hygiene, including handwashing, and to avoid contaminated food and water.

Gastrointestinal infections are a common condition that can cause a range of symptoms from mild to severe. If your child is experiencing symptoms of a gastrointestinal infection,

Motility Disorders

Pediatric motility disorders are conditions that affect the function and movement of the gastrointestinal tract in infants, children, and adolescents. These disorders can cause a range of symptoms, including feeding difficulties, abdominal pain, and constipation. In this answer, we will discuss the common types, symptoms, diagnosis, and treatment of pediatric motility disorders.

Types of Pediatric Motility Disorders:

1. Gastroesophageal Reflux Disease (GERD): GERD is a common condition in which the contents of the stomach back up into the esophagus, causing heartburn and other symptoms.
2. Gastroparesis: Gastroparesis is a condition in which the stomach takes too long to empty its contents into the small intestine, causing nausea, vomiting, and bloating.
3. Intestinal Dysmotility: Intestinal dysmotility refers to a group of conditions that affect the movement of the intestines, causing constipation, diarrhea, and abdominal pain.
4. Hirschsprung's Disease: Hirschsprung's disease is a rare condition in which the nerves that control the movement of the colon do not develop properly, causing constipation and other symptoms.

Symptoms: The symptoms of pediatric motility disorders vary depending on the type and severity of the disorder. Some common symptoms are:

- Feeding difficulties, including poor appetite and weight loss
- Abdominal pain or cramping
- Nausea or vomiting
- Constipation or diarrhea
- Bloating or gas
- Regurgitation or vomiting of food or liquid
- Delayed or prolonged emptying of the stomach
- Failure to thrive

Diagnosis: Pediatric motility disorders are diagnosed based on a combination of medical history, physical examination, and diagnostic tests. The doctor may perform a barium swallow or upper GI series to check for GERD or other abnormalities in the esophagus, stomach, or small intestine. A gastric emptying study may be done to diagnose gastroparesis. In some cases, anorectal manometry or colonic transit studies may be done to diagnose intestinal dysmotility or Hirschsprung's disease.

Treatment: The treatment of pediatric motility disorders depends on the type and severity of the disorder. Some common treatments are:

1. Medications: Certain medications may be prescribed to treat the underlying disorder or symptoms of pediatric motility disorders. For example, prokinetic agents may be prescribed to stimulate the movement of the intestines, and acid reducers may be prescribed to manage GERD.
2. Nutritional Support: Children with pediatric motility disorders may have poor appetite and malnutrition due to poor nutrient absorption. Nutritional support, including specialized diets or supplements, may be required to maintain adequate nutrition.
3. Surgery: In some cases, surgery may be required to treat pediatric motility disorders. For example, surgery may be necessary to remove the affected portion of the colon in children with Hirschsprung's disease.
4. Behavioral Interventions: Behavioral interventions, such as biofeedback or pelvic floor muscle exercises, may be used to treat pediatric motility disorders that affect the rectum or anal sphincter.

Pediatric motility disorders are conditions that can cause a range of symptoms and complications in infants, children, and adolescents.

Intestinal Polyps

Pediatric intestinal polyps are abnormal growths that occur in the intestines of children. These growths may be benign (noncancerous) or malignant (cancerous), and they can occur anywhere in the intestinal tract, including the colon and rectum. In this answer, we will discuss the common types, symptoms, diagnosis, and treatment of pediatric intestinal polyps.

Types of Pediatric Intestinal Polyps:

1. Juvenile Polyps: Juvenile polyps are the most common type of intestinal polyps in children. They are benign growths that occur in the colon or rectum, and they can cause rectal bleeding, diarrhea, and abdominal pain.
2. Peutz-Jeghers Syndrome: Peutz-Jeghers syndrome is a rare genetic disorder that causes multiple intestinal polyps, as well as pigmented spots on the lips, mouth, and other parts of the body. Children with this syndrome may experience abdominal pain, diarrhea, and rectal bleeding.
3. Familial Adenomatous Polyposis (FAP): FAP is a rare genetic disorder that causes the development of numerous adenomatous polyps in the colon and rectum. These polyps have a high risk of developing into cancer, and children with FAP may require surgery to remove the affected portion of the colon.

Symptoms: The symptoms of pediatric intestinal polyps can vary depending on the type, size, and location of the polyp. Some common symptoms are:

- Rectal bleeding
- Abdominal pain or cramping
- Diarrhea or constipation
- Changes in bowel habits
- Anemia or fatigue
- Nausea or vomiting
- Weight loss or poor weight gain

Diagnosis: Pediatric intestinal polyps are diagnosed based on a combination of medical history, physical examination, and diagnostic tests. A colonoscopy or flexible sigmoidoscopy may be performed to visualize the polyps and take a biopsy for further analysis. Blood tests may also be done to check for anemia or other signs of inflammation in the body. Genetic testing may be recommended for children with multiple polyps or a family history of intestinal polyps or cancer.

Treatment: The treatment of pediatric intestinal polyps depends on the type, size, and location of the polyp, as well as the child's age and overall health. Some common treatments are:

1. Polypectomy: Polypectomy is a procedure in which the polyp is removed through a colonoscopy or flexible sigmoidoscopy. This is the preferred treatment for most benign polyps, such as juvenile polyps.
2. Surgery: Surgery may be required to remove large or multiple polyps, or in cases where the polyps have a high risk of developing into cancer. For example, children with FAP may require surgery to remove the affected portion of the colon.
3. Surveillance: Children with a history of intestinal polyps may require regular surveillance to monitor for the development of new polyps or cancer. This may involve regular colonoscopies, blood tests, or imaging studies.
4. Genetic Counseling: Children with genetic disorders, such as Peutz-Jeghers syndrome or FAP, may benefit from genetic counseling and testing to assess their risk of developing polyps or cancer in the future.

Pediatric intestinal polyps are abnormal growths that can occur anywhere in the intestinal tract of children.

Malabsorption Syndromes

Malabsorption syndromes are a group of disorders that affect the ability of the digestive system to properly absorb nutrients from food. Malabsorption can occur due to a variety of reasons, including defects in the lining of the intestines, enzyme deficiencies, and abnormalities in the lymphatic system. In this answer, we will discuss the common types, symptoms, diagnosis, and treatment of pediatric malabsorption syndromes.

Types of Malabsorption Syndromes:

1.   Celiac Disease: Celiac disease is an autoimmune disorder that causes damage to the lining of the small intestine in response to gluten, a protein found in wheat, barley, and rye. This damage can lead to malabsorption of nutrients, and children with celiac disease may experience symptoms such as diarrhea, abdominal pain, and weight loss.

2.   Cystic Fibrosis: Cystic fibrosis is a genetic disorder that affects the production of mucus in the body. This can lead to the production of thick mucus in the pancreas, which can block the flow of digestive enzymes into the small intestine. This can result in malabsorption of nutrients, and children with cystic fibrosis may experience symptoms such as bulky stools, abdominal pain, and weight loss.

3.   Short Bowel Syndrome: Short bowel syndrome is a condition that occurs when a large portion of the small intestine is removed or damaged due to surgery or disease. This can lead to malabsorption of nutrients, and children with short bowel syndrome may experience symptoms such as diarrhea, dehydration, and weight loss.

4.   Lactose Intolerance: Lactose intolerance is a condition that occurs when the body is unable to properly digest lactose, a sugar found in milk and dairy products. This

can lead to malabsorption of nutrients, and children with lactose intolerance may experience symptoms such as diarrhea, bloating, and abdominal pain.

Symptoms: The symptoms of malabsorption syndromes can vary depending on the type and severity of the condition. Some common symptoms are:

- Diarrhea or loose stools
- Abdominal pain or cramping
- Bloating or gas
- Weight loss or poor weight gain
- Fatigue or weakness
- Vitamin or mineral deficiencies
- Delayed growth or development

Diagnosis: Malabsorption syndromes are diagnosed based on a combination of medical history, physical examination, and diagnostic tests. Blood tests may be performed to check for deficiencies in vitamins and minerals, such as iron, calcium, and vitamin B12. Stool tests may also be done to check for the presence of fat or undigested food particles. In some cases, a biopsy of the small intestine may be taken to assess the extent of damage to the intestinal lining.

Treatment: The treatment of malabsorption syndromes depends on the type and severity of the condition, as well as the child's age and overall health. Some common treatments are:

1. Dietary Changes: Dietary changes may be recommended to avoid certain foods or increase the intake of certain nutrients. For example, children with celiac disease may need to avoid gluten, while children with lactose intolerance may need to avoid dairy products.
2. Enzyme Replacement Therapy: Enzyme replacement therapy may be recommended for children with pancreatic enzyme deficiencies, such as those with cystic

fibrosis. This involves taking oral enzyme supplements to aid in the digestion and absorption of nutrients.

3.	Nutritional Support: Nutritional support may be required for children with severe malabsorption or nutrient deficiencies. This may involve intravenous or tube feeding to ensure adequate intake of nutrients.

4.	Medications: Medications may be prescribed to treat specific symptoms, such as diarrhea or abdominal pain.

Malabsorption syndromes can have a significant impact on a child's growth and development. Early recognition and diagnosis of these conditions are essential for appropriate treatment and management. A multidisciplinary approach involving gastroenterologists, nutritionists, and other specialists may be necessary to provide optimal care for children with malabsorption syndromes. With proper treatment and management, most children with malabsorption syndromes can lead normal and healthy lives.

CHAPTER 3

Endocrinology

Pediatric endocrinology is a medical specialty that deals with the diagnosis and treatment of hormonal disorders in children. Some of the common diagnoses that are treated by pediatric endocrinologists include:

1. Type 1 diabetes: This is a condition in which the body is unable to produce enough insulin, which is needed to regulate blood sugar levels.
2. Type 2 diabetes: This is a chronic metabolic disorder characterized by insulin resistance.
3. Growth disorders: These are conditions in which children have abnormal growth patterns, either growing too slowly or too quickly.
4. Thyroid disorders: These are conditions that affect the thyroid gland, which is responsible for regulating metabolism and other functions in the body.
5. Disorders of puberty: These are conditions in which children experience early or delayed puberty, or in which puberty occurs abnormally.
6. Adrenal disorders: These are conditions that affect the adrenal glands, which produce hormones such as cortisol and aldosterone.
7. Disorders of sex development: These are conditions in which the development of the reproductive system is

abnormal, leading to issues with gender identity or sexual development.

8. Calcium and bone disorders: These are conditions that affect the levels of calcium and other minerals in the body, leading to problems with bone growth and development.

9. Pituitary disorders: These are conditions that affect the pituitary gland, which produces hormones that regulate other glands in the body.

10. Hypoglycemia: This is a condition in which blood sugar levels are too low, and can cause symptoms such as dizziness, confusion, and seizures.

11. Hyperlipidemia: This is a condition in which levels of cholesterol and other fats in the blood are too high, increasing the risk of heart disease.

Type 1 Diabetes Mellitus

Type 1 diabetes mellitus (T1DM) is a chronic metabolic disorder characterized by the destruction of insulin-producing beta cells in the pancreas, leading to insulin deficiency and subsequent hyperglycemia. T1DM is most commonly diagnosed in children and adolescents, although it can occur at any age.

Causes: T1DM is caused by a combination of genetic and environmental factors. Genetic susceptibility plays a major role, and children with a family history of T1DM are at a higher risk of developing the disease. Environmental triggers, such as viral infections or exposure to toxins, may also play a role in the development of T1DM.

Symptoms: The classic symptoms of T1DM include frequent urination, increased thirst, increased hunger, weight loss, fatigue, and blurry vision. Children may also experience mood swings, irritability, and difficulty concentrating.

Diagnosis: T1DM diagnosis is based on blood tests that measure blood glucose levels and the presence of autoantibodies that attack the pancreas. The most common autoantibodies associated with T1DM are anti-glutamic acid decarboxylase (GAD) and anti-islet cell antibodies.

Treatment: The primary goal of treatment for T1DM is to maintain blood glucose levels within a normal range to prevent complications. This is achieved through a combination of insulin therapy, blood glucose monitoring, and lifestyle modifications. Insulin therapy involves the use of insulin injections or an insulin pump to provide the body with the insulin it needs. Blood glucose monitoring is essential for adjusting insulin doses and preventing episodes of hypoglycemia or hyperglycemia. Lifestyle modifications, such as a healthy diet and regular exercise, can also help to manage blood glucose levels.

Complications: T1DM can lead to several complications if left untreated or poorly managed. These include:

- Diabetic ketoacidosis (DKA): a potentially life-threatening condition that occurs when the body breaks down fat for energy instead of glucose, leading to high levels of ketones in the blood.
- Hypoglycemia: a condition characterized by low blood glucose levels, which can cause symptoms such as shaking, sweating, and confusion.
- Hyperglycemia: a condition characterized by high blood glucose levels, which can cause long-term complications such as nerve damage, kidney damage, and eye damage.
- Cardiovascular disease: T1DM increases the risk of developing cardiovascular disease, including heart attacks and strokes.
- Neuropathy: T1DM can damage the nerves, leading to numbness, tingling, and other sensations in the limbs.

Prevention: Currently, there is no known way to prevent T1DM. However, researchers are investigating strategies to delay or prevent the onset of the disease in high-risk individuals, such as those with a family history of T1DM.

Type 2 Diabetes Mellitus

Type 2 diabetes mellitus (T2DM) is a chronic metabolic disorder characterized by insulin resistance, which means that the body's cells do not respond properly to insulin. T2DM is typically diagnosed in children and adolescents who are overweight or obese and have a family history of the disease.

Causes: The exact cause of T2DM is not fully understood, but it is believed to be caused by a combination of genetic and environmental factors. Children with a family history of T2DM, or those who are overweight or obese and lead a sedentary lifestyle, are at an increased risk of developing the disease.

Symptoms: The symptoms of T2DM in children are similar to those in adults and may include increased thirst, frequent urination, blurred vision, fatigue, and slow healing of wounds. Children may also have no symptoms at all, which can make diagnosis more difficult.

Diagnosis: The diagnosis of T2DM in children is based on blood tests that measure blood glucose levels and other markers of insulin resistance. These tests may include a fasting glucose test, an oral glucose tolerance test, and a hemoglobin A1C test.

Treatment: The primary goal of treatment for T2DM is to control blood glucose levels to prevent complications. This is achieved through a combination of lifestyle modifications, such as weight loss, healthy eating habits, and regular exercise, and medication. Medications may include oral antidiabetic medications or insulin therapy, depending on the severity of

the disease.
Complications:

T2DM can lead to several complications if left untreated or poorly managed. These include:

- Cardiovascular disease: T2DM increases the risk of developing cardiovascular disease, including heart attacks and strokes.
- Kidney damage: T2DM can damage the kidneys over time, leading to a condition called diabetic nephropathy.
- Eye damage: T2DM can damage the blood vessels in the eyes, leading to a condition called diabetic retinopathy.
- Nerve damage: T2DM can damage the nerves, leading to numbness, tingling, and other sensations in the limbs.

Prevention: The best way to prevent T2DM in children is through healthy lifestyle habits, such as a balanced diet and regular physical activity. Parents can encourage their children to eat a healthy diet rich in fruits, vegetables, and whole grains and limit sugary and high-fat foods. Encouraging regular physical activity and limiting sedentary behaviors, such as excessive screen time, can also help prevent T2DM in children.

Growth Disorders

Pediatric growth disorders refer to conditions that affect the normal growth and development of children. These disorders can affect various aspects of growth, such as height, weight, and bone development. Some of the common pediatric growth disorders include:

1. Growth hormone deficiency (GHD): GHD is a condition where the body does not produce enough growth hormone, which is essential for normal growth and development. Children with GHD may have delayed growth, short stature, and slow development of muscle

mass and bone density.

2.   Turner syndrome: Turner syndrome is a genetic disorder that affects females and results in the absence of all or part of one X chromosome. Children with Turner syndrome may have short stature, delayed puberty, and other physical abnormalities such as a webbed neck, a low hairline, and abnormal ears.

3.   Achondroplasia: Achondroplasia is a genetic disorder that affects bone growth, resulting in short stature, disproportionately short limbs, and a large head with a prominent forehead.

4.   Hypothyroidism: Hypothyroidism is a condition where the thyroid gland does not produce enough thyroid hormone, which is essential for normal growth and development. Children with hypothyroidism may have delayed growth, slow development, and other symptoms such as fatigue, constipation, and dry skin.

5.   Prader-Willi syndrome: Prader-Willi syndrome is a genetic disorder that affects various aspects of growth and development, including low muscle tone, delayed growth and puberty, and an insatiable appetite that can lead to obesity.

6.   Klinefelter syndrome is a genetic condition that occurs when a male is born with an extra X chromosome, resulting in a karyotype of 47,XXY instead of the typical male karyotype of 46,XY.

Growth Hormone Deficiency

Pediatric growth hormone deficiency (GHD) is a medical condition characterized by insufficient secretion of growth hormone (GH) from the pituitary gland, which can lead to poor growth and development in children. GH plays a vital role in stimulating growth and development in children, including bone growth, muscle development, and organ growth.

The causes of GHD can vary and may include genetic disorders, brain tumors or injuries, infections, autoimmune diseases, and certain medications. Children with GHD may present with symptoms such as short stature, delayed growth, delayed puberty, low bone density, and reduced muscle mass. Additionally, children with GHD may experience other health problems such as increased body fat, reduced strength and endurance, and a decreased quality of life.

Diagnosis of GHD involves a thorough medical history and physical examination, as well as specialized tests such as a GH stimulation test, insulin-like growth factor-1 (IGF-1) measurement, and imaging studies such as magnetic resonance imaging (MRI) of the brain.

Treatment for GHD typically involves growth hormone replacement therapy, which involves injecting synthetic growth hormone into the body to stimulate growth and development. Treatment is usually initiated as soon as possible to prevent or reduce the negative effects of GHD on growth and development. Treatment typically continues until the child has reached their final adult height or until their growth plates have closed.

In addition to growth hormone replacement therapy, children with GHD may benefit from additional treatments such as nutritional and lifestyle interventions, medications to treat related health conditions such as osteoporosis, and psychological support to help cope with the emotional and social challenges of the condition.

Turner Syndrome

Turner syndrome is a genetic disorder that affects females

and is caused by a missing or abnormal X chromosome. It is estimated to affect approximately 1 in 2,500 female births. Females with Turner syndrome often experience a wide range of physical and developmental problems, which can vary in severity depending on the individual.

The symptoms of Turner syndrome can include short stature, low hairline at the back of the neck, a webbed neck, low-set ears, swollen hands and feet, and a broad chest with widely spaced nipples. Affected individuals may also experience hormonal imbalances, including a lack of ovarian function, which can result in infertility and amenorrhea (absent or irregular menstrual periods). Additionally, individuals with Turner syndrome may experience learning difficulties, hearing and vision problems, and heart and kidney defects.

Diagnosis of Turner syndrome is typically made through a karyotype analysis, which is a genetic test that examines an individual's chromosomes to identify any abnormalities. The test involves taking a sample of the individual's blood or other tissues, and then examining the cells for any missing or abnormal X chromosomes.

Treatment for Turner syndrome typically involves addressing the individual symptoms associated with the condition. For example, hormone replacement therapy may be used to replace the hormones that are not produced by the ovaries, and growth hormone therapy may be used to help improve height. Additionally, individuals with Turner syndrome may require surgery to correct certain physical abnormalities, such as aortic coarctation (a narrowing of the aorta) or kidney malformations.

Turner syndrome is a genetic disorder that affects females and is caused by a missing or abnormal X chromosome. It can result in a wide range of physical and developmental problems, which can vary in severity depending on the individual.

Treatment typically involves addressing the individual symptoms associated with the condition, and may include hormone replacement therapy, growth hormone therapy, and surgery. Early diagnosis and management of Turner syndrome can help improve outcomes and quality of life for affected individuals.

Achondroplasia

Achondroplasia is a genetic disorder that affects bone growth, resulting in short stature and other physical features. It is the most common form of dwarfism, with an incidence of approximately 1 in 25,000 births.

Achondroplasia is caused by a mutation in the fibroblast growth factor receptor 3 (FGFR3) gene, which regulates bone growth. The mutation leads to abnormal bone growth in the arms, legs, and spine, resulting in shortened limbs, a large head with a prominent forehead, and a flattened bridge of the nose. Additionally, individuals with achondroplasia may experience health problems such as obesity, sleep apnea, and spinal stenosis.

Diagnosis of achondroplasia can be made prenatally through ultrasound imaging, or after birth through physical examination and genetic testing. Treatment for achondroplasia is aimed at managing the symptoms associated with the condition, and may include monitoring for health problems such as spinal stenosis or sleep apnea, and interventions such as surgery to correct spinal abnormalities.

In addition to medical treatment, individuals with achondroplasia may benefit from early intervention services such as physical therapy, occupational therapy, and speech therapy to address developmental delays and promote optimal growth and development. Educational support and psychological counseling may also be helpful to address the emotional and social challenges associated with living with achondroplasia.

Achondroplasia is a genetic disorder that affects bone growth, resulting in short stature and other physical features. Diagnosis can be made prenatally or after birth through physical examination and genetic testing. Treatment for achondroplasia is aimed at managing the symptoms associated with the condition, and may include monitoring for health problems and interventions such as surgery. Early intervention services, educational support, and psychological counseling may also be helpful for affected individuals and their families.

Congenital Hypothyroidism

Congenital hypothyroidism (CH) is a medical condition in which a newborn baby has an underactive thyroid gland, leading to low levels of thyroid hormone in the body. This can result in a wide range of physical and developmental problems if left untreated.

The thyroid gland is a butterfly-shaped gland located in the neck that produces hormones essential for growth, development, and metabolism. In CH, the thyroid gland either does not develop properly or does not produce enough thyroid hormone. The condition is typically diagnosed through newborn screening tests, which are performed shortly after birth.

Symptoms of CH can include prolonged jaundice, poor feeding, constipation, decreased muscle tone, lethargy, and delayed growth and development. If left untreated, CH can lead to severe intellectual disability, growth failure, hearing loss, and other complications.

Treatment for CH involves replacing the missing thyroid

hormone with a synthetic thyroid hormone called levothyroxine. The medication is typically given daily as an oral tablet, and must be continued for life. Regular monitoring of thyroid hormone levels is necessary to ensure that the correct dose is being administered and to adjust the dose as needed.

Early diagnosis and treatment of CH are essential to prevent long-term complications and ensure optimal growth and development. Newborn screening programs have been implemented in many countries to detect CH and other conditions early, allowing for prompt treatment and improved outcomes.

Congenital hypothyroidism is a medical condition in which a newborn baby has an underactive thyroid gland, leading to low levels of thyroid hormone in the body. Symptoms can include prolonged jaundice, poor feeding, constipation, lethargy, and delayed growth and development. Treatment involves replacing the missing thyroid hormone with a synthetic hormone called levothyroxine, which must be continued for life. Early diagnosis and treatment are essential to prevent long-term complications and ensure optimal growth and development.

Prader-Willi Syndrome

Prader-Willi syndrome (PWS) is a rare genetic disorder that affects approximately 1 in 10,000 to 1 in 30,000 individuals. It is caused by a genetic defect on chromosome 15 that results in a wide range of physical, behavioral, and cognitive symptoms.

The symptoms of PWS can vary widely, but most individuals with the condition have weak muscle tone, delayed development, and poor feeding during infancy. As they grow older, they may develop an insatiable appetite and an intense craving for food, leading to obesity and related health problems. Other symptoms of PWS can include intellectual disability, short stature, delayed puberty, behavioral problems, sleep disturbances, and difficulty regulating body temperature.

PWS is typically diagnosed through genetic testing, which can identify the genetic defect on chromosome 15. Treatment for PWS is aimed at managing the symptoms associated with the condition, and may include a combination of medication, dietary interventions, and behavioral therapy.

One of the most important aspects of treatment for PWS is managing the individual's diet to prevent obesity and related health problems. This may involve restricting caloric intake and providing a balanced, nutrient-rich diet. In some cases, growth hormone therapy may also be used to help improve growth and development.

Behavioral therapy may also be helpful for individuals with PWS, particularly in managing the behavioral and emotional problems associated with the condition. This may include cognitive-behavioral therapy, social skills training, and parent training to help parents and caregivers manage challenging behaviors.

Prader-Willi syndrome is a rare genetic disorder that affects physical, behavioral, and cognitive development. It is caused by a genetic defect on chromosome 15 and is typically diagnosed through genetic testing. Treatment for PWS is aimed at managing the symptoms associated with the condition, and may include medication, dietary interventions, and behavioral therapy. Managing the individual's diet is particularly important to prevent obesity and related health problems. Early diagnosis and treatment are essential to help individuals with PWS achieve their full potential and lead fulfilling lives.

Klinefelter Syndrome

Klinefelter syndrome is a genetic condition that occurs when a male is born with an extra X chromosome, resulting in a karyotype of 47,XXY instead of the typical male karyotype of 46,XY. This extra X chromosome can cause a wide range of physical, cognitive, and developmental symptoms.

Some of the physical symptoms of Klinefelter syndrome can include tall stature, long limbs, gynecomastia (enlarged breast tissue), small testes, and reduced facial and body hair. Individuals with Klinefelter syndrome may also have an increased risk of health problems such as osteoporosis, type 2 diabetes, and autoimmune disorders.

Cognitive and developmental symptoms of Klinefelter syndrome can vary widely, but may include learning difficulties, speech and language delays, social and emotional difficulties, and behavioral problems. Some individuals with Klinefelter syndrome may also have difficulties with motor skills and coordination.

Diagnosis of Klinefelter syndrome can be made through genetic testing, which can identify the extra X chromosome. Treatment for Klinefelter syndrome is aimed at managing the symptoms associated with the condition, and may include hormone replacement therapy (such as testosterone replacement therapy) to address low testosterone levels, speech and language therapy, and educational interventions to address learning difficulties.

Early diagnosis and treatment of Klinefelter syndrome is important to prevent or manage the physical and cognitive symptoms associated with the condition. With appropriate management, individuals with Klinefelter syndrome can lead fulfilling lives and achieve their full potential.

Klinefelter syndrome is a genetic condition that occurs when a male is born with an extra X chromosome, resulting in a range of physical, cognitive, and developmental symptoms. Diagnosis is typically made through genetic testing, and treatment may include hormone replacement therapy, speech and language therapy, and educational interventions. Early diagnosis and management is important to help individuals with Klinefelter syndrome achieve their full potential.

Thyroid Disorders

Pediatric thyroid disorders refer to conditions that affect the thyroid gland in children. The thyroid gland produces hormones that are essential for normal growth and development, metabolism, and overall health. Thyroid disorders can affect children of all ages, from infants to adolescents. Some of the common pediatric thyroid disorders include:

1. Congenital hypothyroidism: Congenital hypothyroidism is a condition where the thyroid gland does not produce enough thyroid hormone at birth. If left untreated, it can result in delayed growth and development, intellectual disability, and other complications.

2. Hyperthyroidism: Hyperthyroidism is a condition where the thyroid gland produces too much thyroid hormone. Children with hyperthyroidism may experience weight loss, rapid heartbeat, increased appetite, nervousness, and other symptoms.

3. Hypothyroidism: Hypothyroidism is a condition where the thyroid gland does not produce enough thyroid hormone. Children with hypothyroidism may experience weight gain, fatigue, cold intolerance, constipation, and other symptoms.

4. Hashimoto's thyroiditis: Hashimoto's thyroiditis is an autoimmune disorder that causes inflammation of the

thyroid gland. Over time, this can lead to hypothyroidism.

5.   Thyroid nodules: Thyroid nodules are growths or lumps that form in the thyroid gland. Most thyroid nodules in children are benign, but in rare cases, they can be cancerous.

6.   Graves' disease: This is a type of autoimmune disorder that affects the thyroid gland, which is located in the neck and produces hormones that regulate metabolism

Congenital Hypothyroidism (CH)

Congenital hypothyroidism (CH) is a medical condition in which a newborn baby has an underactive thyroid gland, leading to low levels of thyroid hormone in the body. This can result in a wide range of physical and developmental problems if left untreated.

The thyroid gland is a butterfly-shaped gland located in the neck that produces hormones essential for growth, development, and metabolism. In CH, the thyroid gland either does not develop properly or does not produce enough thyroid hormone. The condition is typically diagnosed through newborn screening tests, which are performed shortly after birth.

Symptoms of CH can include prolonged jaundice, poor feeding, constipation, decreased muscle tone, lethargy, and delayed growth and development. If left untreated, CH can lead to severe intellectual disability, growth failure, hearing loss, and other complications.

Treatment for CH involves replacing the missing thyroid hormone with a synthetic thyroid hormone called levothyroxine. The medication is typically given daily as an oral tablet, and must be continued for life. Regular monitoring of thyroid hormone levels is necessary to ensure that the correct dose is being administered and to adjust the dose as needed.

Early diagnosis and treatment of CH are essential to prevent long-term complications and ensure optimal growth and development. Newborn screening programs have been implemented in many countries to detect CH and other conditions early, allowing for prompt treatment and improved outcomes.

Congenital hypothyroidism is a medical condition in which a newborn baby has an underactive thyroid gland, leading to low levels of thyroid hormone in the body. Symptoms can include prolonged jaundice, poor feeding, constipation, lethargy, and delayed growth and development. Treatment involves replacing the missing thyroid hormone with a synthetic hormone called levothyroxine, which must be continued for life. Early diagnosis and treatment are essential to prevent long-term complications and ensure optimal growth and development.

Hyperthyroidism

Hyperthyroidism is a rare condition that occurs when the thyroid gland in children produces too much thyroid hormone. This can cause a wide range of physical and cognitive symptoms.

Some of the physical symptoms of hyperthyroidism can include weight loss, increased appetite, rapid heartbeat, sweating, heat intolerance, tremors, and fatigue. Children with hyperthyroidism may also experience an enlarged thyroid gland, called a goiter. In some cases, hyperthyroidism can cause eye problems such as bulging eyes or eye irritation.

Cognitive symptoms of hyperthyroidism can include difficulty concentrating, irritability, anxiety, and mood swings. In severe cases, hyperthyroidism can cause psychosis or delirium.

Diagnosis of hyperthyroidism is typically made through a combination of physical examination, blood tests, and imaging tests such as an ultrasound or scan of the thyroid gland. Treatment for pediatric hyperthyroidism may include medication to reduce thyroid hormone levels, radioactive iodine therapy to shrink the thyroid gland, or surgery to remove part or all of the thyroid gland.

In addition to these treatments, children with hyperthyroidism may also benefit from dietary interventions such as increasing their intake of calcium and vitamin D to prevent bone loss, and avoiding caffeine and other stimulants that can exacerbate symptoms.

Long-term management of hyperthyroidism is important to prevent complications such as bone loss, heart problems, and eye problems. With appropriate treatment and management, most children with hyperthyroidism can lead healthy and fulfilling lives.

Hyperthyroidism is a rare condition that occurs when the thyroid gland produces too much thyroid hormone in children. Symptoms can include physical and cognitive changes, and diagnosis is typically made through a combination of physical examination and medical tests. Treatment may include medication, radioactive iodine therapy, or surgery, and dietary interventions may also be recommended. Long-term management is important to prevent complications and ensure a healthy and fulfilling life.

Hypothyroidism

Hypothyroidism is a condition that occurs when the thyroid gland in children produces too little thyroid hormone. This can cause a wide range of physical and cognitive symptoms.

Some of the physical symptoms of hypothyroidism can include weight gain, fatigue, dry skin, constipation, cold intolerance, hair loss, and a hoarse voice. Children with hypothyroidism may also have an enlarged thyroid gland, called a goiter. In some cases, hypothyroidism can cause delayed growth and development, as well as delayed onset of puberty.

Cognitive symptoms of hypothyroidism can include difficulty concentrating, poor memory, and depression. In severe cases, hypothyroidism can cause intellectual disability or developmental delays.

Diagnosis of hypothyroidism is typically made through a combination of physical examination, blood tests to measure thyroid hormone levels, and imaging tests such as an ultrasound or scan of the thyroid gland. Treatment for pediatric hypothyroidism typically involves hormone replacement therapy, in which children are given a synthetic form of the thyroid hormone to make up for the deficiency.

Children with hypothyroidism may also benefit from dietary interventions such as increasing their intake of iodine and avoiding foods that can interfere with the absorption of thyroid hormone. Additionally, children with hypothyroidism may be at risk for other health problems such as high cholesterol and anemia, and may require additional monitoring and treatment for these conditions.

Long-term management of hypothyroidism is important to ensure healthy growth and development, and to prevent complications such as heart problems and intellectual disability. With appropriate treatment and management, most children with hypothyroidism can lead healthy and fulfilling lives.

Hypothyroidism is a condition that occurs when the thyroid

gland produces too little thyroid hormone in children, causing a range of physical and cognitive symptoms. Diagnosis is typically made through a combination of physical examination and medical tests, and treatment involves hormone replacement therapy. Children with hypothyroidism may also benefit from dietary interventions and may require additional monitoring for other health problems. Long-term management is important to ensure healthy growth and development and prevent complications.

Hashimoto's Thyroiditis

Hashimoto's thyroiditis is an autoimmune disorder that affects the thyroid gland, which is responsible for producing thyroid hormones that regulate metabolism. In Hashimoto's thyroiditis, the immune system attacks the thyroid gland, leading to inflammation and damage. This damage can result in reduced thyroid function, leading to hypothyroidism.

Hashimoto's thyroiditis is more common in women and can occur at any age, but it most commonly affects middle-aged women. It may also occur in children, although it is less common. The cause of Hashimoto's thyroiditis is not completely understood, but it is thought to be a combination of genetic and environmental factors.

Symptoms of Hashimoto's thyroiditis can vary, but typically include fatigue, weight gain, sensitivity to cold, dry skin, constipation, joint pain, and depression. Children may also experience delayed growth and puberty. In some cases, the thyroid gland may enlarge, causing a visible lump in the neck.

Diagnosis of Hashimoto's thyroiditis is typically made through blood tests that measure thyroid hormone levels and the presence of antibodies that target the thyroid gland. An ultrasound of the thyroid gland may also be used to evaluate the size and appearance of the gland.

Treatment for Hashimoto's thyroiditis typically involves hormone replacement therapy, in which patients are given a synthetic form of the thyroid hormone to make up for the deficiency. The dosage of the hormone replacement therapy is adjusted based on blood tests and clinical symptoms. In some cases, the thyroid gland may need to be removed surgically if it is causing significant symptoms or if there is a risk of cancer.

In addition to hormone replacement therapy, some dietary and lifestyle changes may be helpful for patients with Hashimoto's thyroiditis. These may include avoiding foods that can interfere with thyroid function, such as soy, and increasing intake of foods that contain iodine, a nutrient that is essential for thyroid function. Exercise and stress-reduction techniques may also be helpful for managing symptoms.

Hashimoto's thyroiditis is an autoimmune disorder that affects the thyroid gland, causing inflammation and damage that can result in hypothyroidism. Diagnosis is typically made through blood tests and imaging tests, and treatment involves hormone replacement therapy and possibly surgery. Dietary and lifestyle changes may also be helpful for managing symptoms. With appropriate treatment and management, most patients with Hashimoto's thyroiditis can lead healthy and fulfilling lives.

Thyroid Nodules

Thyroid nodules are lumps or growths that develop within the thyroid gland, which is located in the neck and produces hormones that regulate metabolism. Most thyroid nodules are benign (non-cancerous) and do not cause any symptoms, but in some cases, they can lead to overproduction of thyroid hormone (hyperthyroidism) or compress nearby structures, causing symptoms such as difficulty swallowing or breathing.

Thyroid nodules are common, and many people may have them without realizing it. Risk factors for developing thyroid nodules include age (they are more common in older individuals), being female, having a family history of thyroid nodules or thyroid cancer, and exposure to radiation.

Diagnosis of thyroid nodules typically involves a physical examination of the neck, blood tests to measure thyroid hormone levels, and imaging tests such as ultrasound, CT scan, or MRI to visualize the nodule and assess its size and characteristics. In some cases, a biopsy may be performed to determine if the nodule is cancerous.

Treatment for thyroid nodules depends on several factors, including the size and characteristics of the nodule, whether or not it is causing symptoms, and whether it is cancerous. Small nodules that are not causing any symptoms may not require any treatment, but regular monitoring may be recommended to ensure they do not grow or become cancerous. In cases where the nodule is causing symptoms or is at risk for being cancerous, surgery may be necessary to remove all or part of the thyroid gland.

In some cases, thyroid nodules may be treated with radioactive iodine therapy or hormone suppression therapy, which involves taking synthetic thyroid hormones to suppress the production of thyroid-stimulating hormone (TSH) and shrink the nodule.

Thyroid nodules are lumps or growths that develop within the thyroid gland and can be either benign or cancerous. Diagnosis typically involves physical examination, blood tests, and imaging tests, and treatment depends on the size, characteristics, and symptoms of the nodule. Most thyroid nodules are benign and do not require treatment, but regular monitoring is often recommended to ensure they do not grow or become cancerous.

Graves' Disease

Graves' disease is a type of autoimmune disorder that affects the thyroid gland, which is located in the neck and produces hormones that regulate metabolism. In Graves' disease, the immune system produces antibodies that cause the thyroid gland to produce too much thyroid hormone, leading to hyperthyroidism.

Graves' disease is more common in females and has a genetic component, with a higher risk for those with a family history of the condition. Symptoms can vary but may include:

- Rapid or irregular heartbeat
- Nervousness or irritability
- Weight loss
- Increased sweating and intolerance to heat
- Muscle weakness or tremors
- Enlarged thyroid gland (goiter)
- Bulging eyes (ophthalmopathy)

Diagnosis of Graves' disease involves a physical examination, blood tests to measure thyroid hormone levels and antibodies, and imaging tests such as ultrasound or radioactive iodine uptake scan to visualize the thyroid gland and assess its function. A biopsy may also be performed to rule out other conditions.

Treatment for Graves' disease may involve medication, radioactive iodine therapy, or surgery. Medications such as antithyroid drugs, beta blockers, or steroids can help to manage symptoms and slow down the production of thyroid hormone. Radioactive iodine therapy involves taking a pill or liquid containing radioactive iodine, which is taken up by the thyroid gland and destroys the cells that produce thyroid hormone. Surgery may be recommended in severe cases or if other treatments are not effective.

In addition to medical treatment, lifestyle changes such as reducing stress, getting regular exercise, and eating a healthy diet may also be recommended to help manage symptoms and support overall health.

Graves' disease is an autoimmune disorder that causes hyperthyroidism and is characterized by symptoms such as rapid heartbeat, nervousness, and weight loss. Diagnosis involves a physical examination, blood tests, and imaging tests, and treatment may involve medication, radioactive iodine therapy, or surgery. Lifestyle changes may also be recommended to manage symptoms and support overall health.

Disorders of Puberty

Pediatric disorders of puberty refer to conditions that affect the normal onset and progression of puberty in children. Puberty is a complex process that involves the activation of the hypothalamic-pituitary-gonadal axis, which leads to the development of secondary sexual characteristics, growth spurt, and hormonal changes. Disorders of puberty can affect various aspects of this process, leading to delayed or premature puberty, abnormal sexual development, and other complications. Some of the common pediatric disorders of puberty include:

1.   Precocious puberty: Precocious puberty is a condition where puberty starts too early, usually before the age of 8 in girls and 9 in boys. Children with precocious puberty may develop breast tissue, pubic hair, and other secondary sexual characteristics at a younger age than normal.

2.   Delayed puberty: Delayed puberty is a condition where puberty starts later than normal, usually after the age

of 14 in boys and 13 in girls. Children with delayed puberty may have slower growth, delayed development of secondary sexual characteristics, and other symptoms.

3. Hypogonadism: Hypogonadism is a condition where the gonads (ovaries in females and testes in males) do not produce enough sex hormones. This can lead to delayed puberty, incomplete sexual development, and other complications.

4. Turner syndrome: Turner syndrome is a genetic disorder that affects females and results in the absence of all or part of one X chromosome. Children with Turner syndrome may have delayed puberty, short stature, and other physical abnormalities such as a webbed neck and abnormal ears.

5. Klinefelter syndrome: Klinefelter syndrome is a genetic disorder that affects males and results in the presence of an extra X chromosome. Children with Klinefelter syndrome may have delayed puberty, incomplete sexual development, and other symptoms such as tall stature, reduced muscle mass, and gynecomastia (breast tissue development).

Precocious Puberty

Precocious puberty is a condition in which a child experiences the onset of puberty earlier than the usual age range. It is more common in girls than in boys and can occur as early as age 6 in girls and age 9 in boys.

The signs of precocious puberty in girls may include the development of breast buds, the growth of pubic and underarm hair, and the onset of menstruation. In boys, signs may include testicular growth and the growth of pubic, underarm, and facial hair. Children with precocious puberty may also experience a growth spurt and develop adult body odor earlier than their peers.

There are two types of precocious puberty: central precocious puberty and peripheral precocious puberty. Central precocious puberty, also known as gonadotropin-dependent precocious puberty, is caused by the premature activation of the hypothalamic-pituitary-gonadal axis, which regulates the release of sex hormones. Peripheral precocious puberty, also known as gonadotropin-independent precocious puberty, is caused by the production of sex hormones by the adrenal glands or other organs outside of the hypothalamic-pituitary-gonadal axis.

The causes of precocious puberty can vary and may be genetic or related to other medical conditions such as tumors, infections, or hormonal imbalances. In some cases, the cause may be unknown.

Treatment for precocious puberty may involve medication to delay the onset of puberty and slow the progression of sexual development. Gonadotropin-releasing hormone (GnRH) analogs, such as leuprolide, are commonly used to suppress the release of sex hormones and delay the onset of puberty. In some cases, surgery may be necessary to remove tumors or other growths that are causing precocious puberty.

In addition to medical treatment, children with precocious puberty may benefit from psychological support to help them cope with the emotional and social challenges that can arise from early sexual development.

Precocious puberty is a condition in which a child experiences the onset of puberty earlier than the usual age range. It can be caused by a variety of factors and is treated with medication or surgery to delay the onset of puberty and slow the progression of sexual development. Psychological support may also be beneficial for children with precocious puberty.

Delayed Puberty

Delayed puberty is a condition in which puberty does not begin at the usual age range. In girls, delayed puberty is defined as the absence of breast development by age 13 or the absence of menstruation by age 16. In boys, delayed puberty is defined as the absence of testicular enlargement by age 14.

There are many potential causes of delayed puberty, including genetic factors, hormonal imbalances, chronic illness, malnutrition, and certain medications. In some cases, the cause may be unknown.

The diagnosis of delayed puberty typically involves a physical exam and blood tests to evaluate hormone levels. Imaging studies, such as X-rays, may also be done to assess bone age, which can help determine the likelihood of puberty starting in the near future.

Treatment for delayed puberty depends on the underlying cause. In some cases, no treatment may be necessary, as puberty may start on its own at a later age. However, if there is a hormonal imbalance or other medical condition causing delayed puberty, treatment may be necessary. For example, if a deficiency in growth hormone or thyroid hormone is identified, replacement therapy may be prescribed. If the delay is due to a problem with the hypothalamus or pituitary gland, medication may be prescribed to stimulate hormone production.

In some cases, children with delayed puberty may experience emotional or social challenges due to their delayed physical development. They may benefit from counseling or support groups to help them cope with these challenges and develop a positive body image.

Delayed puberty is a condition in which puberty does not

begin at the usual age range. It can have a variety of potential causes and may require treatment depending on the underlying condition. Children with delayed puberty may benefit from counseling or support to help them cope with the emotional and social challenges that can arise from delayed physical development.

Hypogonadism

Hypogonadism is a medical condition in which the gonads (ovaries or testes) produce little or no sex hormones. This can result in a variety of symptoms depending on the age and gender of the individual affected.

In males, hypogonadism can present as delayed puberty, decreased libido, erectile dysfunction, decreased muscle mass and strength, fatigue, and mood changes. In severe cases, it can also lead to osteoporosis, infertility, and increased risk of cardiovascular disease.

In females, hypogonadism can present as delayed puberty, amenorrhea (absence of menstrual periods), decreased libido, infertility, and osteoporosis.

There are two main types of hypogonadism: primary and secondary. Primary hypogonadism occurs when the gonads themselves are not functioning properly. This can be due to genetic factors, injury, radiation or chemotherapy treatment, infection, or autoimmune disease. Secondary hypogonadism occurs when there is a problem with the hypothalamus or pituitary gland, which are responsible for signaling the gonads to produce sex hormones. Causes of secondary hypogonadism can include tumors, injury, radiation, infection, or congenital defects.

The diagnosis of hypogonadism typically involves blood tests to measure hormone levels, including testosterone and estrogen. Imaging studies, such as ultrasound or MRI, may also be done to evaluate the gonads and pituitary gland.

Treatment for hypogonadism depends on the underlying cause and can involve hormone replacement therapy (HRT) with testosterone or estrogen. In some cases, HRT may be administered in the form of patches, gels, injections, or pellets. Lifestyle changes, such as diet and exercise, may also be recommended to manage symptoms and improve overall health.

Hypogonadism is a medical condition in which the gonads produce little or no sex hormones, resulting in a range of symptoms depending on age and gender. Primary and secondary hypogonadism are the two main types, with different underlying causes and treatment options. A proper diagnosis and individualized treatment plan can help manage symptoms and improve overall health.

Turner Syndrome

Turner syndrome is a genetic disorder that affects females and is caused by a missing or abnormal X chromosome. It is estimated to affect approximately 1 in 2,500 female births. Females with Turner syndrome often experience a wide range of physical and developmental problems, which can vary in severity depending on the individual.

The symptoms of Turner syndrome can include short stature, low hairline at the back of the neck, a webbed neck, low-set ears, swollen hands and feet, and a broad chest with widely spaced nipples. Affected individuals may also experience hormonal imbalances, including a lack of ovarian function, which can result in infertility and amenorrhea (absent or irregular menstrual periods). Additionally, individuals with Turner syndrome may experience learning difficulties, hearing and vision problems, and heart and kidney defects.

Diagnosis of Turner syndrome is typically made through a karyotype analysis, which is a genetic test that examines an individual's chromosomes to identify any abnormalities. The test involves taking a sample of the individual's blood or other tissues, and then examining the cells for any missing or abnormal X chromosomes.

Treatment for Turner syndrome typically involves addressing the individual symptoms associated with the condition. For example, hormone replacement therapy may be used to replace the hormones that are not produced by the ovaries, and growth hormone therapy may be used to help improve height. Additionally, individuals with Turner syndrome may require surgery to correct certain physical abnormalities, such as aortic coarctation (a narrowing of the aorta) or kidney malformations.

Turner syndrome is a genetic disorder that affects females and is caused by a missing or abnormal X chromosome. It can result in a wide range of physical and developmental problems, which can vary in severity depending on the individual. Treatment typically involves addressing the individual symptoms associated with the condition, and may include hormone replacement therapy, growth hormone therapy, and surgery. Early diagnosis and management of Turner syndrome can help improve outcomes and quality of life for affected individuals.

Adrenal Disorders

Adrenal disorders refer to conditions that affect the adrenal glands in children. The adrenal glands are two small glands located on top of the kidneys that produce hormones that are essential for regulating metabolism, blood pressure, stress response, and other bodily functions. Adrenal disorders can affect children of all ages, from infants to adolescents. Some of the common pediatric adrenal disorders include:

1. Congenital adrenal hyperplasia (CAH): CAH is a group of genetic disorders that affect the production of adrenal hormones. Children with CAH may have salt wasting, ambiguous genitalia, and other symptoms.

2. Adrenal insufficiency: Adrenal insufficiency is a condition where the adrenal glands do not produce enough hormones. Children with adrenal insufficiency may experience fatigue, weight loss, low blood pressure, and other symptoms.

3. Cushing's syndrome: Cushing's syndrome is a condition where the adrenal glands produce too much cortisol hormone. Children with Cushing's syndrome may experience weight gain, high blood pressure, mood changes, and other symptoms.

4. Adrenocortical carcinoma: Adrenocortical carcinoma is a rare form of cancer that affects the adrenal glands. Children with this condition may experience abdominal pain, weight loss, and other symptoms.

5. Pheochromocytoma: Pheochromocytoma is a rare tumor that develops in the adrenal glands and can produce excess amounts of adrenaline and noradrenaline hormones. Children with pheochromocytoma may experience high blood pressure, headaches, and other symptoms

Congenital Adrenal Hyperplasia (CAH)

Congenital adrenal hyperplasia (CAH) is a group of genetic disorders that affect the adrenal glands, which are responsible for producing steroid hormones. These disorders are caused by mutations in genes involved in the production of these hormones, resulting in the overproduction of androgens (male sex hormones) and the underproduction of cortisol (a stress hormone) and aldosterone (a hormone that regulates salt and water balance).

The most common form of CAH is caused by a deficiency of the enzyme 21-hydroxylase, which is involved in the production of cortisol and aldosterone. Without this enzyme, the adrenal glands produce excess androgens, leading to virilization (masculinization) of the external genitalia in female fetuses and precocious (early) puberty in both males and females. This can also lead to other symptoms such as excessive body hair growth, acne, menstrual irregularities, infertility, and short stature.

Diagnosis of CAH typically involves measuring hormone levels in blood or urine and may also involve genetic testing. Prenatal diagnosis is also possible through chorionic villus sampling or amniocentesis.

Treatment for CAH involves replacing deficient hormones (cortisol and aldosterone) and reducing the production of androgens. This is typically achieved through steroid replacement therapy, which involves daily administration of synthetic cortisol and sometimes also aldosterone. The goal is to maintain normal hormone levels and prevent excess androgen production, thereby minimizing the risk of virilization or early puberty. Regular monitoring of hormone levels and growth is important to adjust the dosage of hormone replacement therapy as needed.

Congenital adrenal hyperplasia is a group of genetic disorders that affect the production of steroid hormones, resulting in excess androgen production and deficient cortisol and aldosterone production. The most common form is caused by a deficiency of the enzyme 21-hydroxylase. Treatment involves hormone replacement therapy to replace deficient hormones and reduce androgen production. Early diagnosis and treatment are important to prevent complications and optimize growth and development.

Adrenal Insufficiency

Adrenal insufficiency is a medical condition where the adrenal glands, located on top of the kidneys, fail to produce enough of the hormones cortisol and aldosterone. Cortisol helps regulate metabolism and the body's response to stress, while aldosterone helps maintain the body's salt and water balance.

There are two types of adrenal insufficiency: primary and secondary. Primary adrenal insufficiency, also known as Addison's disease, is caused by damage to the adrenal glands themselves, usually due to autoimmune disorders, infections, or cancer. Secondary adrenal insufficiency is caused by a problem with the pituitary gland or hypothalamus, which regulate the production of cortisol and aldosterone.

Symptoms of adrenal insufficiency can vary depending on the severity of the condition and the underlying cause. Common symptoms include fatigue, weakness, weight loss, loss of appetite, abdominal pain, nausea, vomiting, low blood pressure, and darkening of the skin.

Diagnosis of adrenal insufficiency involves a physical examination, blood tests to measure hormone levels, and stimulation tests to evaluate the adrenal glands' response to stress. Imaging tests, such as computed tomography (CT) or magnetic resonance imaging (MRI), may also be done to check for any damage or abnormalities in the adrenal glands.

Treatment for adrenal insufficiency involves replacing the deficient hormones with synthetic cortisol and sometimes aldosterone. This is typically done through oral medications or injections. The dosage and timing of the medication may need to be adjusted based on the patient's hormone levels and response to treatment.

In cases of primary adrenal insufficiency, patients may also need to take medications to suppress the immune system or undergo surgery to remove any cancerous or damaged adrenal glands. In cases of secondary adrenal insufficiency, treatment may involve addressing the underlying problem with the pituitary gland or hypothalamus.

Adrenal insufficiency is a medical condition where the adrenal glands fail to produce enough cortisol and aldosterone. It can be caused by damage to the adrenal glands themselves or a problem with the pituitary gland or hypothalamus. Treatment involves replacing the deficient hormones with synthetic cortisol and sometimes aldosterone, along with addressing any underlying causes or complications. Early diagnosis and treatment are important to prevent potentially life-threatening complications.

Cushing's Syndrome

Cushing's syndrome is a rare endocrine disorder caused by prolonged exposure to high levels of cortisol, a hormone produced by the adrenal glands. It can also be caused by excessive use of corticosteroid medications. Cortisol helps regulate metabolism and the body's response to stress.

There are two main types of Cushing's syndrome: endogenous and exogenous. Endogenous Cushing's syndrome is caused by the body producing too much cortisol, usually due to a tumor on the pituitary gland or adrenal gland, or rarely, elsewhere in the body. Exogenous Cushing's syndrome is caused by taking high doses of corticosteroid medications over a long period of time.

Symptoms of Cushing's syndrome can vary depending on the underlying cause and the severity of the condition. Common symptoms include weight gain, especially in the upper body and face, muscle weakness, fatigue, thinning of the skin, easy bruising, high blood pressure, and mood changes.

Diagnosis of Cushing's syndrome involves a physical examination, blood and urine tests to measure cortisol levels, and imaging tests such as computed tomography (CT) or magnetic resonance imaging (MRI) to look for tumors or other abnormalities in the adrenal gland or pituitary gland. Additional tests such as a dexamethasone suppression test, in which a synthetic steroid is given to see how the body responds, may also be done.

Treatment for Cushing's syndrome depends on the underlying cause. In cases of endogenous Cushing's syndrome, surgery may be needed to remove the tumor causing the excess cortisol production. In some cases, radiation therapy or medications to block cortisol production may be used. In cases of exogenous Cushing's syndrome, gradually reducing the dose of corticosteroid medications or switching to a different medication may be necessary.

Complications of Cushing's syndrome can include increased risk of infections, high blood pressure, diabetes, osteoporosis, and mood disorders. With proper treatment, most people with Cushing's syndrome can recover and manage their symptoms effectively.

Cushing's syndrome is a rare endocrine disorder caused by prolonged exposure to high levels of cortisol, either due to the body producing too much cortisol or excessive use of corticosteroid medications. Symptoms can vary and diagnosis involves physical examination, blood and urine tests, and imaging tests. Treatment depends on the underlying cause and can involve surgery, radiation therapy, or medications.

Complications can occur, but most people with Cushing's syndrome can manage their symptoms with proper treatment.

Adrenocortical Carcinoma

Adrenocortical carcinoma (ACC) is a rare type of cancer that develops in the adrenal gland, which is located on top of the kidneys. ACC is a type of endocrine tumor, meaning that it produces hormones, usually in excess. The adrenal gland produces several hormones, including cortisol, aldosterone, and androgens, which regulate metabolism, blood pressure, and sexual development.

The exact cause of ACC is unknown, but some cases may be linked to genetic mutations or inherited conditions such as Li-Fraumeni syndrome or Beckwith-Wiedemann syndrome. Other risk factors include exposure to radiation or certain chemicals.

Symptoms of ACC depend on the hormones being produced by the tumor. The most common symptom is abdominal pain, often with a mass or swelling in the abdomen. Other symptoms may include weight gain, muscle weakness, high blood pressure, irregular periods or early puberty in females, and signs of virilization (excessive growth of facial or body hair, deepening of the voice) in females and males.

Diagnosis of ACC involves a combination of imaging tests, blood tests to check hormone levels, and a biopsy to confirm the presence of cancer cells. Imaging tests may include computed tomography (CT), magnetic resonance imaging (MRI), or positron emission tomography (PET) scans.

Treatment for ACC usually involves surgery to remove the tumor and possibly the entire affected adrenal gland. Radiation therapy and chemotherapy may also be used to treat the cancer, especially if it has spread to other parts of the body. Medications may be used to manage symptoms caused by excess hormone production.

The prognosis for ACC depends on the stage of the cancer, the size and location of the tumor, and the patient's overall health. Early diagnosis and treatment can lead to a better prognosis. However, because ACC is a rare and aggressive cancer, it often spreads to other parts of the body before it is diagnosed, making it difficult to treat.

Adrenocortical carcinoma is a rare and aggressive cancer that develops in the adrenal gland and is often linked to excess hormone production. Symptoms depend on the hormones being produced and may include abdominal pain, weight gain, muscle weakness, high blood pressure, and signs of virilization. Diagnosis involves a combination of imaging tests, blood tests, and a biopsy. Treatment may involve surgery, radiation therapy, chemotherapy, and medications. The prognosis for ACC depends on several factors, including the stage of the cancer, the size and location of the tumor, and the patient's overall health.

Pheochromocytoma

Pheochromocytoma is a rare type of tumor that originates in the adrenal glands, which are located on top of the kidneys. The tumor produces excessive amounts of hormones called catecholamines, which regulate the body's response to stress. The majority of pheochromocytomas are benign, but they can also be malignant.

The exact cause of pheochromocytoma is unknown, but it is believed to be related to genetic mutations. The tumor can occur in individuals of any age, but it is more commonly found in adults between the ages of 30 and 60.

Symptoms of pheochromocytoma are caused by excess catecholamines and can vary depending on the level of hormone production. Common symptoms include high blood pressure, headache, sweating, rapid heartbeat, palpitations, anxiety, and weight loss. In severe cases, patients may experience chest pain, shortness of breath, or even heart failure.

Diagnosis of pheochromocytoma involves a combination of imaging tests, blood tests, and a urine test to measure the level of catecholamines and their byproducts. Imaging tests such as computed tomography (CT) or magnetic resonance imaging (MRI) can help locate the tumor.

Treatment for pheochromocytoma involves surgical removal of the tumor. Prior to surgery, medications may be used to control blood pressure and heart rate, as these can be elevated due to the excess catecholamines. After surgery, regular monitoring is necessary to ensure that the tumor does not recur.

Pheochromocytoma is a rare tumor that originates in the adrenal glands and produces excessive amounts of hormones called catecholamines. Symptoms include high blood pressure, headache, sweating, and anxiety. Diagnosis involves a combination of imaging tests, blood tests, and a urine test. Treatment involves surgical removal of the tumor, with medications used to control symptoms prior to surgery. Regular monitoring is necessary to ensure that the tumor does not recur.

Disorders of Sex Development

Pediatric disorders of sex development (DSD) refer to a group of conditions where there is a mismatch between the chromosomal, gonadal, and anatomical sex of a child. These disorders can affect various aspects of sexual development, including the development of internal and external genitalia, hormonal balance, and reproductive function. Some of the common pediatric DSD include:

1. Congenital adrenal hyperplasia (CAH): CAH is a group of genetic disorders that affect the production of adrenal hormones. This can lead to abnormal genitalia in females and early onset of puberty in both sexes.

2. Androgen insensitivity syndrome (AIS): AIS is a genetic disorder where the body is unable to respond to male sex hormones (androgens). This can lead to incomplete development of male sexual characteristics in males and female genitalia in females.

3. Turner syndrome: Turner syndrome is a genetic disorder that affects females and results in the absence of all or part of one X chromosome. Children with Turner syndrome may have incomplete sexual development, short stature, and other physical abnormalities such as a webbed neck and abnormal ears.

4. Klinefelter syndrome: Klinefelter syndrome is a genetic disorder that affects males and results in the presence of an extra X chromosome. Children with Klinefelter syndrome may have incomplete sexual development, reduced muscle mass, and other symptoms.

5. Gonadal dysgenesis: Gonadal dysgenesis is a genetic disorder where the gonads (ovaries in females and testes in males) do not develop properly. This can lead to incomplete sexual development, infertility, and other complications.

Androgen Insensitivity Syndrome

Androgen insensitivity syndrome (AIS) is a genetic disorder

that affects sexual development in individuals with XY chromosomes (typically males). AIS occurs when the body is unable to respond properly to androgens, which are hormones that promote the development of male sex characteristics. As a result, individuals with AIS have some or all of the physical characteristics of a female, despite having male chromosomes.

There are three types of AIS: complete, partial, and mild. In complete AIS, the body is unable to respond to androgens, so the individual develops physical characteristics of a female, such as breasts and a female pattern of pubic hair. The external genitalia may appear female or ambiguous. Internal structures, such as testes and a shortened vagina, are also present.

In partial AIS, the body is partially able to respond to androgens, resulting in a wide range of physical characteristics, including ambiguous genitalia, a smaller-than-average penis, and testes that may be undescended or located in the abdomen. Mild AIS is the mildest form of the condition, and the individual has mostly male physical characteristics, but may have breast development and sparse pubic hair.

AIS is caused by a mutation in the androgen receptor gene, which is located on the X chromosome. The severity of the condition depends on the type and location of the mutation.

Diagnosis of AIS typically occurs during childhood, when parents or doctors may notice that a child with male chromosomes is not developing male physical characteristics. Diagnostic tests may include hormone testing, genetic testing, and imaging studies.

Treatment for AIS depends on the severity of the condition and the individual's personal preferences. In many cases, surgery may be recommended to remove testes and/or create a more female-like appearance of the external genitalia.

Hormone therapy may also be used to promote breast development and feminine fat distribution.

Androgen insensitivity syndrome is a genetic disorder that affects sexual development in individuals with male chromosomes. The severity of the condition depends on the type and location of the mutation. Diagnosis typically occurs during childhood, and treatment may include surgery and hormone therapy.

Turner Syndrome

Turner syndrome is a genetic disorder that affects females and is caused by a missing or abnormal X chromosome. It is estimated to affect approximately 1 in 2,500 female births. Females with Turner syndrome often experience a wide range of physical and developmental problems, which can vary in severity depending on the individual.

The symptoms of Turner syndrome can include short stature, low hairline at the back of the neck, a webbed neck, low-set ears, swollen hands and feet, and a broad chest with widely spaced nipples. Affected individuals may also experience hormonal imbalances, including a lack of ovarian function, which can result in infertility and amenorrhea (absent or irregular menstrual periods). Additionally, individuals with Turner syndrome may experience learning difficulties, hearing and vision problems, and heart and kidney defects.

Diagnosis of Turner syndrome is typically made through a karyotype analysis, which is a genetic test that examines an individual's chromosomes to identify any abnormalities. The test involves taking a sample of the individual's blood or other tissues, and then examining the cells for any missing or abnormal X chromosomes.

Treatment for Turner syndrome typically involves addressing the individual symptoms associated with the condition. For example, hormone replacement therapy may be used to replace the hormones that are not produced by the ovaries, and growth hormone therapy may be used to help improve height. Additionally, individuals with Turner syndrome may require surgery to correct certain physical abnormalities, such as aortic coarctation (a narrowing of the aorta) or kidney malformations.

Turner syndrome is a genetic disorder that affects females and is caused by a missing or abnormal X chromosome. It can result in a wide range of physical and developmental problems, which can vary in severity depending on the individual. Treatment typically involves addressing the individual symptoms associated with the condition, and may include hormone replacement therapy, growth hormone therapy, and surgery. Early diagnosis and management of Turner syndrome can help improve outcomes and quality of life for affected individuals.

Gonadal Dysgenesis

Gonadal dysgenesis is a rare genetic disorder that affects the development of the gonads, which are the organs responsible for producing gametes (eggs or sperm) and sex hormones. In individuals with gonadal dysgenesis, the gonads do not develop properly, leading to infertility and other medical issues.

There are several different types of gonadal dysgenesis, including pure gonadal dysgenesis, mixed gonadal dysgenesis, and Swyer syndrome. Pure gonadal dysgenesis occurs when the gonads do not develop at all, leading to infertility and a lack of sex hormone production. Mixed gonadal dysgenesis occurs when the gonads develop abnormally, leading to a mixture of testicular and ovarian tissue. Swyer syndrome is a type of mixed gonadal dysgenesis that is caused by a mutation in the SRY gene, which is responsible for the development of male sex characteristics.

Symptoms of gonadal dysgenesis can vary depending on the type of the disorder, but may include delayed puberty, infertility, absence of menstruation, ambiguous genitalia, and other physical abnormalities.

Diagnosis of gonadal dysgenesis typically involves genetic testing and imaging studies to evaluate the gonads and other reproductive structures. Treatment may involve surgery to remove the abnormal gonads and hormone therapy to promote the development of secondary sex characteristics and prevent bone loss.

Individuals with gonadal dysgenesis are at an increased risk of developing certain medical conditions, such as osteoporosis, cardiovascular disease, and certain cancers. Therefore, it is important for individuals with gonadal dysgenesis to receive regular medical monitoring and screening for these conditions.

Gonadal dysgenesis is a rare genetic disorder that affects the development of the gonads, leading to infertility and other medical issues. Diagnosis typically involves genetic testing and imaging studies, and treatment may involve surgery and hormone therapy. Individuals with gonadal dysgenesis are at an increased risk of developing certain medical conditions and should receive regular medical monitoring and screening.

Calcium and Bone Disorders

Calcium and bone disorders refer to a group of conditions that affect the development, growth, and maintenance of bones in children. These conditions can result in a variety of bone-related problems such as brittle bones, curvature of the spine, stunted growth, and other complications. Some of the common pediatric calcium and bone disorders include:

1. Rickets: Rickets is a condition where there is a deficiency of vitamin D, calcium, or phosphate, which can lead to softening and weakening of bones. This can cause bone deformities, stunted growth, and other complications.

2. Osteogenesis imperfecta (OI): OI is a genetic disorder where there is a defect in the production of collagen, a protein that is essential for bone strength. Children with OI may have brittle bones that are prone to fractures, as well as hearing loss and other complications.

3. Juvenile idiopathic arthritis (JIA): JIA is an autoimmune disorder that affects the joints, causing inflammation and damage to the bones. This can lead to joint stiffness, pain, and deformity, as well as growth problems in some children.

4. Hyperparathyroidism: Hyperparathyroidism is a condition where there is excessive secretion of parathyroid hormone, which can lead to bone loss, weakened bones, and other complications.

5. Osteoporosis: Osteoporosis is a condition where there is a loss of bone density, making bones weak and fragile. This can increase the risk of fractures and other complications.

Diagnosis of calcium and bone disorders typically involves a combination of physical exams, medical history review, and diagnostic tests such as blood tests, imaging studies, and bone density testing. Treatment for these disorders will depend on the underlying cause and may include medications, hormone therapy, lifestyle changes, and surgery.

Calcium and bone disorders are a group of conditions that can affect the development, growth, and maintenance of bones in children. These disorders can be caused by various factors, including nutritional deficiencies, genetic abnormalities, hormonal imbalances, and environmental factors. Early diagnosis and treatment of these disorders can help prevent or minimize bone-related complications and ensure that affected children achieve optimal growth and development.

Rickets

Rickets is a condition that affects the bones of growing children, causing them to become weak and soft. Rickets is usually caused by a deficiency in vitamin D, calcium, or phosphorus, which are essential nutrients for bone health.

Symptoms of rickets can include delayed growth, bowing of the legs, thickened wrists and ankles, and pain or tenderness in the bones. Children with rickets may also be at an increased risk of developing fractures and dental problems.

The most common cause of rickets is a lack of exposure to sunlight, which is necessary for the body to produce vitamin D. Other causes can include a diet low in vitamin D, calcium, or phosphorus, certain medical conditions that affect nutrient absorption or metabolism, and certain medications.

Diagnosis of rickets typically involves a physical exam, blood tests to measure levels of vitamin D, calcium, and phosphorus, and X-rays to evaluate the bones. Treatment may involve vitamin D and/or calcium supplements, increased sun exposure, and dietary changes to ensure adequate nutrient intake. In severe cases, braces or surgery may be necessary to correct bone deformities.

Prevention of rickets involves ensuring that children receive adequate levels of vitamin D and other essential nutrients through a healthy diet and/or supplements, and exposure to sunlight. Infants who are exclusively breastfed may be at a higher risk of developing rickets and may require vitamin D supplements.

Rickets is a condition that affects the bones of growing children, typically caused by a deficiency in vitamin D, calcium, or phosphorus. Symptoms can include delayed growth, bone deformities, and pain or tenderness in the bones. Diagnosis involves a physical exam, blood tests, and X-rays, and treatment may involve supplements, sun exposure, and dietary changes. Prevention involves ensuring adequate nutrient intake and exposure to sunlight.

Osteogenesis Imperfecta

Osteogenesis imperfecta (OI), also known as brittle bone disease, is a rare genetic disorder characterized by bones that are fragile and easily broken. OI affects the body's ability to produce collagen, a protein that gives structure to bones, skin, and other connective tissues.

There are four main types of OI, ranging in severity from mild to severe. The most common type is Type I, which is the mildest form and typically causes bones to fracture easily. Type II is the most severe form and is often fatal, as infants born with this condition have very weak bones that can break in utero or during delivery. Types III and IV are intermediate in severity.

Symptoms of OI can include frequent fractures, bone deformities, short stature, and loose joints. People with OI may also experience hearing loss, dental problems, and breathing difficulties. In severe cases, OI can lead to disability and a shortened lifespan.

Diagnosis of OI typically involves a physical exam, genetic testing, and imaging studies such as X-rays or bone density scans. Treatment for OI is focused on managing symptoms and preventing fractures. This may involve medications to strengthen bones, physical therapy to improve mobility and strength, and surgery to correct bone deformities or repair fractures.

People with OI may also benefit from assistive devices such as braces, wheelchairs, or other mobility aids. In some cases, gene therapy or other experimental treatments may be available.

While there is no cure for OI, ongoing research is focused on developing new treatments and improving outcomes for people with the condition. Early diagnosis and intervention can help improve quality of life and prevent complications associated with OI.

Juvenile Idiopathic Arthritis (JIA)

Juvenile idiopathic arthritis (JIA) is a chronic autoimmune disease that affects children and adolescents, typically under the age of 16. It is the most common form of arthritis in children.

JIA is characterized by inflammation of the joints, which can cause pain, swelling, stiffness, and limited mobility. The disease can also affect other parts of the body, such as the eyes, skin, and internal organs.

There are several types of JIA, each with its own set of symptoms and disease course. These include:

1. Oligoarticular JIA: This is the most common type of JIA, affecting four or fewer joints in the first six months of the disease.
2. Polyarticular JIA: This type of JIA affects five or more joints within the first six months of the disease. It can be further divided into two subtypes: rheumatoid factor-positive and rheumatoid factor-negative.
3. Systemic JIA: This is the most serious type of JIA, as it can affect internal organs in addition to the joints. Children with systemic JIA may experience fever, rash, and other symptoms in addition to joint pain and swelling.
4. Enthesitis-related JIA: This type of JIA is characterized by inflammation where tendons and ligaments attach to

bone, causing pain and swelling in the joints.

The exact cause of JIA is unknown, but it is believed to involve a combination of genetic and environmental factors. There is no cure for JIA, but treatment can help manage symptoms and prevent joint damage.

Treatment options for JIA include:

1. Nonsteroidal anti-inflammatory drugs (NSAIDs) to reduce pain and inflammation
2. Disease-modifying antirheumatic drugs (DMARDs) to slow the progression of the disease
3. Biologic drugs to target specific aspects of the immune system
4. Physical therapy to improve joint mobility and strength
5. Occupational therapy to help children with JIA perform daily activities
6. Joint injections with steroids or other medications to reduce inflammation
7. Surgery in severe cases to repair or replace damaged joints.

Early diagnosis and treatment of JIA can help prevent joint damage and improve long-term outcomes. Children with JIA may also benefit from ongoing support from a multidisciplinary team of healthcare professionals, including pediatric rheumatologists, physical therapists, and occupational therapists.

Hyperparathyroidism

Hyperparathyroidism is a rare endocrine disorder in children that is characterized by excessive secretion of parathyroid hormone (PTH) from the parathyroid glands. This results in elevated serum calcium levels (hypercalcemia) and decreased phosphate levels (hypophosphatemia), which can lead to a variety of clinical manifestations.

There are two types of hyperparathyroidism in children: primary and secondary. Primary hyperparathyroidism (PHPT) is caused by a benign tumor in one or more of the parathyroid glands, while secondary hyperparathyroidism (SHPT) is a compensatory response to hypocalcemia or vitamin D deficiency.

Symptoms of hyperparathyroidism in children can vary depending on the age of onset, severity of hypercalcemia, and duration of the disease. Some common symptoms include:

- Abdominal pain
- Anorexia
- Nausea and vomiting
- Constipation
- Frequent urination
- Dehydration
- Fatigue
- Muscle weakness
- Bone pain or fractures
- Growth failure or short stature
- Cognitive impairment

In severe cases, hypercalcemia can lead to cardiac arrhythmias, kidney stones, and renal failure.

The diagnosis of hyperparathyroidism in children is based on laboratory tests including serum calcium, phosphate, PTH, and 25-hydroxyvitamin D levels. Imaging studies such as ultrasound, sestamibi scan, or MRI may also be performed to localize the parathyroid adenoma.

Treatment of hyperparathyroidism in children depends on the type and severity of the disease. In PHPT, surgical removal of the affected parathyroid gland(s) is the definitive treatment. In SHPT, treatment focuses on correcting the underlying condition causing the hypocalcemia or vitamin D deficiency, such as supplementation with calcium and vitamin D. Bisphosphonate therapy may also be used to reduce bone resorption and prevent fractures.

Long-term follow-up is important for children with hyperparathyroidism to monitor for potential complications such as recurrent hypercalcemia, nephrocalcinosis, and osteoporosis.

Osteoporosis

Osteoporosis is a rare condition characterized by reduced bone density and increased susceptibility to fractures in children and adolescents. The diagnosis of osteoporosis in children is usually made based on the presence of a fragility fracture and reduced bone density on dual-energy X-ray absorptiometry (DXA) scan.

Causes: There are several causes of osteoporosis, including genetic disorders, hormonal imbalances, chronic diseases, and certain medications. Some of the common causes include:

1. Genetic disorders: Several genetic disorders such as osteogenesis imperfecta, Marfan syndrome, and Ehlers-Danlos syndrome can cause pediatric osteoporosis.
2. Hormonal imbalances: Hormonal imbalances such as hyperthyroidism, hyperparathyroidism, and Cushing's syndrome can lead to bone loss and osteoporosis.
3. Chronic diseases: Chronic diseases such as inflammatory bowel disease, celiac disease, and chronic kidney disease can affect bone health and increase the risk of osteoporosis.
4. Medications: Certain medications such as glucocorticoids, anticonvulsants, and immunosuppressants can cause osteoporosis in children.

Symptoms: Osteoporosis is often asymptomatic, and the first sign may be a fracture. Fractures may occur with minimal or no trauma, and the affected bone may be painful, tender, and swollen. The fractures most commonly occur in the spine, hip, and wrist. Children with severe osteoporosis may also have short stature, skeletal deformities, and delayed puberty.

Treatment: The treatment of osteoporosis involves identifying and treating the underlying cause, if possible. Children with osteoporosis should be advised to maintain a healthy lifestyle, including regular exercise and a diet rich in calcium and vitamin D. Calcium and vitamin D supplements may also be recommended to improve bone health.

In some cases, medication may be necessary to prevent further bone loss and reduce the risk of fractures. Bisphosphonates are the most commonly used medications for pediatric osteoporosis, although their safety and efficacy in children are not well established.

In severe cases of osteoporosis, bone marrow transplantation may be considered. However, this is a risky and complicated procedure and is usually reserved for severe and life-threatening cases.

The prognosis for osteoporosis depends on the underlying cause, severity of the disease, and the effectiveness of treatment. Children with osteoporosis require ongoing monitoring and management to prevent complications and ensure optimal bone health.

Pituitary Disorders

Pediatric pituitary disorders refer to a group of conditions that affect the pituitary gland, a small gland located at the base of the brain that is responsible for producing and regulating various hormones. These disorders can result in a range of hormonal imbalances and related health problems in children. Some of the common pediatric pituitary disorders include:

1. Growth hormone deficiency (GHD): GHD is a condition where there is a lack of production or secretion of growth hormone, which can lead to stunted growth and other complications.

2. Central precocious puberty (CPP): CPP is a condition where there is premature onset of puberty, which can result in early development of sexual characteristics and other complications.

3. Pituitary tumors: Pituitary tumors are abnormal growths in the pituitary gland that can cause hormonal imbalances and other complications. These tumors can be benign or malignant and can affect various hormones, depending on their location and type.

4. Diabetes insipidus (DI): DI is a condition where there is a lack of production or secretion of antidiuretic hormone (ADH), which can lead to excessive thirst and urination.

5. Cushing's syndrome: Cushing's syndrome is a condition where there is excessive secretion of cortisol, a hormone produced by the adrenal glands. This can lead to a range of complications such as weight gain, high blood pressure, and diabetes.

Diagnosis of pediatric pituitary disorders typically involves a combination of physical exams, medical history review, and diagnostic tests such as blood tests, imaging studies, and hormone level measurements. Treatment for these disorders will depend on the underlying cause and may include medications, hormone therapy, surgery, and other interventions.

Pediatric pituitary disorders are a group of conditions that can affect the pituitary gland, leading to hormonal imbalances and related health problems in children. These disorders can be caused by various factors, including genetic abnormalities, tumors, infections, and other medical conditions. Early diagnosis and treatment of these disorders can help prevent or minimize hormonal imbalances and ensure that affected children achieve optimal growth and development.

Growth Hormone Deficiency

Pediatric growth hormone deficiency (PGHD) is a condition characterized by insufficient production of growth hormone (GH) during childhood and adolescence, resulting in growth failure and short stature. The disorder affects approximately 1 in 3,500 to 1 in 10,000 children, and it can be caused by various factors, including genetic mutations, brain injury, and certain medical treatments.

Symptoms of PGHD typically include slow growth and delayed development, resulting in short stature that is often below the 3rd percentile for age and sex. Other symptoms may include a chubby body build, delayed puberty, a high-pitched voice, and weakened bones. Children with PGHD may also experience psychological symptoms, such as social isolation, low self-esteem, and depression, due to their short stature.

The diagnosis of PGHD is typically made through a combination of medical history, physical examination, and laboratory testing. Growth hormone stimulation tests, which measure the body's response to GH injections, are commonly used to confirm the diagnosis.

The treatment of PGHD involves daily injections of synthetic GH to stimulate growth and development. GH therapy has been shown to improve growth rates, increase final adult height, and improve bone density in children with PGHD. The duration of treatment depends on the individual's response to GH therapy and their rate of growth. Treatment may continue until the child reaches their final adult height, which may not occur until the late teenage years or early adulthood.

Complications of PGHD may include an increased risk of cardiovascular disease, reduced bone density, and impaired glucose tolerance. Therefore, children with PGHD require regular monitoring and management of their overall health and wellbeing.

Growth hormone deficiency is a relatively common disorder that can significantly affect a child's growth and development. With early diagnosis and appropriate treatment with GH therapy, children with PGHD can achieve normal or near-normal growth and development, leading to improved quality of life and overall health outcomes.

Central Precocious Puberty (CPP)

Pediatric central precocious puberty (CPP) is a condition characterized by the premature activation of the hypothalamic-pituitary-gonadal axis, resulting in the onset of puberty before the age of 8 years in girls and 9 years in boys. The typical signs of puberty, such as breast development in girls and testicular enlargement in boys, occur earlier than normal. CPP is more common in girls than in boys, and it affects about 1 in 5,000 to 10,000 children.

The causes of CPP are not always clear, but in some cases, it may be due to an underlying medical condition, such as a tumor or a genetic disorder. Other potential causes include exposure to hormones or environmental toxins, obesity, and certain medications.

The diagnosis of CPP typically involves a physical examination, which may reveal signs of puberty, as well as blood tests to measure hormone levels. Imaging studies, such as an MRI of the brain, may be performed to identify any underlying abnormalities that may be causing CPP.

Treatment for CPP typically involves medications to slow or

stop the premature activation of the hypothalamic-pituitary-gonadal axis. These medications include gonadotropin-releasing hormone (GnRH) agonists, which suppress the release of gonadotropins, hormones that stimulate the ovaries or testes to produce sex hormones. Treatment is usually continued until the child reaches an appropriate age for the onset of puberty.

Untreated precocious puberty can lead to psychological distress, short stature, and reduced adult height due to premature closure of the growth plates. Early treatment of CPP can prevent these complications and help affected children achieve normal growth and development.

Pituitary Tumors

Pediatric pituitary tumors are rare, accounting for less than 10% of all pediatric brain tumors. The pituitary gland is a small gland located at the base of the brain, responsible for secreting hormones that control growth and development, metabolism, reproduction, and stress response. Pituitary tumors can either be benign or malignant and can cause an overproduction or underproduction of hormones.

The symptoms of pediatric pituitary tumors can vary depending on the age of the child and the hormones affected. Some common symptoms include headaches, vision changes, nausea and vomiting, fatigue, weight gain, growth delay, early or delayed puberty, excessive thirst and urination, and abnormal menstruation.

Diagnosis of pediatric pituitary tumors involves a thorough medical history, physical examination, and laboratory tests to assess hormone levels. Imaging tests such as magnetic resonance imaging (MRI) and computed tomography (CT) scans are also used to identify the presence and location of the tumor.

Treatment options for pediatric pituitary tumors depend on the type, size, and location of the tumor as well as the severity of the symptoms. In some cases, observation and monitoring may be recommended if the tumor is small and not causing significant symptoms. Surgical removal of the tumor is often necessary for larger or malignant tumors. Radiation therapy and medications that block the production or effects of hormones may also be used in conjunction with surgery.

Early detection and treatment of pediatric pituitary tumors are critical in preventing long-term complications and improving the quality of life for affected children.

Diabetes Insipidus

Diabetes insipidus (DI) is a rare condition in children characterized by the inability of the kidneys to conserve water, resulting in excessive urination and thirst. There are two main types of diabetes insipidus: central diabetes insipidus (CDI) and nephrogenic diabetes insipidus (NDI).

Central diabetes insipidus occurs when the body doesn't produce enough antidiuretic hormone (ADH), also known as vasopressin. This hormone helps to regulate the amount of water in the body by signaling the kidneys to conserve water when needed. In CDI, the lack of ADH production causes the kidneys to excrete large amounts of diluted urine, leading to dehydration, excessive thirst, and frequent urination. CDI can be caused by a variety of factors, including genetic mutations, head trauma, brain tumors, infections, or autoimmune disorders.

Nephrogenic diabetes insipidus, on the other hand, occurs

when the kidneys are unable to respond to ADH, despite normal production levels of the hormone. This can be due to a genetic mutation, medications (such as lithium), kidney disease, or other factors. NDI presents similar symptoms to CDI, including excessive thirst and urination, but is often less severe and can be managed with lifestyle modifications and medication.

The diagnosis of diabetes insipidus in children involves a combination of medical history, physical exam, and laboratory tests. Blood tests may be conducted to measure levels of ADH and other hormones, while urine tests can help evaluate kidney function. Additional imaging studies, such as MRI or CT scans, may also be ordered to check for abnormalities in the brain or kidneys.

Treatment for diabetes insipidus typically involves addressing the underlying cause and managing symptoms. In CDI, replacement therapy with synthetic ADH (desmopressin) may be used to help regulate water balance in the body. In NDI, medications such as thiazide diuretics or nonsteroidal anti-inflammatory drugs (NSAIDs) may be prescribed to help the kidneys respond better to ADH. In severe cases, hospitalization may be required to administer intravenous fluids and medications.

Children with diabetes insipidus require ongoing monitoring and management to ensure proper hydration and prevent complications such as dehydration or electrolyte imbalances. With appropriate treatment and management, children with diabetes insipidus can lead healthy, normal lives.

Cushing's Syndrome

Cushing's syndrome is a rare disorder caused by an excess of cortisol, a hormone that regulates the body's metabolism and immune response. In children, Cushing's syndrome is most commonly caused by the use of high-dose glucocorticoids for the treatment of conditions such as asthma, inflammatory bowel disease, and autoimmune disorders. However, it can also be caused by a tumor in the pituitary gland, adrenal gland, or other parts of the body.

Symptoms of pediatric Cushing's syndrome may include weight gain, particularly in the face, neck, and trunk; high blood pressure; acne; increased body hair growth; delayed growth and development; and a rounded "moon" face. Children may also experience mood changes, including irritability, anxiety, and depression, and may have trouble concentrating or remembering things.

Diagnosis of pediatric Cushing's syndrome involves a physical exam, blood tests to measure cortisol levels, and imaging tests such as a CT scan or MRI to identify any tumors that may be causing the excess cortisol production. In some cases, a sample of urine may also be collected to measure cortisol levels.

Treatment for pediatric Cushing's syndrome typically involves the gradual withdrawal of glucocorticoid medications, if they are the cause of the condition. In cases where a tumor is causing the excess cortisol production, surgery to remove the tumor may be necessary. Radiation therapy or medication to block the production of cortisol may also be used in some cases.

Children with Cushing's syndrome may require ongoing monitoring to ensure that cortisol levels remain within a normal range and to check for any signs of recurrence. It is also important to address any psychological or developmental issues that may have arisen as a result of the condition, such as growth delays or behavioral changes.

Hypoglycemia

Pediatric hypoglycemia refers to a condition where the blood glucose levels in children drop below the normal range, which can lead to a range of symptoms and complications. Hypoglycemia can occur in children with and without diabetes and can result from various factors such as insulin overdose, delayed or missed meals, and underlying medical conditions.

The symptoms of hypoglycemia in children can vary depending on the severity of the condition and the age of the child. Common symptoms include sweating, trembling, confusion, irritability, dizziness, headache, and blurred vision. In severe cases, hypoglycemia can lead to seizures, loss of consciousness, and even coma.

The diagnosis of pediatric hypoglycemia involves measuring blood glucose levels using a glucose meter or laboratory tests. Treatment for hypoglycemia typically involves consuming foods or drinks that are high in glucose or taking medications that can help raise blood sugar levels. If hypoglycemia is caused by an underlying medical condition, treating the underlying condition is necessary.

Prevention of hypoglycemia in children involves ensuring that they eat balanced meals at regular intervals and monitor blood glucose levels if they have diabetes. Children with diabetes are at a higher risk of hypoglycemia and should follow a strict treatment plan that includes insulin injections or other medications as prescribed by their healthcare provider.

Pediatric hypoglycemia is a condition where blood glucose levels in children drop below the normal range, leading to a range of symptoms and complications. Early diagnosis and treatment of hypoglycemia are important to prevent complications and ensure that affected children achieve optimal health and development. Prevention of hypoglycemia involves following a healthy diet, monitoring blood glucose levels regularly, and adhering to a strict treatment plan if the child has diabetes.

Hyperlipidemia

Pediatric hyperlipidemia is a condition where there are high levels of lipids (fats) in the blood in children. Elevated lipid levels in children can lead to an increased risk of developing cardiovascular diseases such as heart attacks and stroke later in life. The most common types of lipids involved in pediatric hyperlipidemia include low-density lipoprotein (LDL) cholesterol and triglycerides.

Pediatric hyperlipidemia can be caused by various factors such as genetics, poor diet, lack of physical activity, and underlying medical conditions such as obesity and diabetes. The condition can also be acquired through certain medications such as corticosteroids and retinoids.

Diagnosis of pediatric hyperlipidemia involves measuring the levels of lipids in the blood using a lipid profile test. The test measures levels of total cholesterol, LDL cholesterol, high-density lipoprotein (HDL) cholesterol, and triglycerides. If the results of the lipid profile test indicate elevated lipid levels, further tests may be necessary to determine the underlying cause of the condition.

Treatment for pediatric hyperlipidemia involves lifestyle modifications and medication therapy. Lifestyle modifications include a healthy diet, regular exercise, and weight management. The American Academy of Pediatrics recommends that children with elevated lipid levels follow a diet that is low in saturated fat and cholesterol and high in fruits, vegetables, and whole grains. Medication therapy may be necessary for children with severe hyperlipidemia or those who do not respond to lifestyle modifications. The most common medications used to treat hyperlipidemia in children include statins, bile acid sequestrants, and niacin.

Prevention of pediatric hyperlipidemia involves encouraging healthy eating habits and physical activity from a young age. Children should be encouraged to consume a healthy diet and engage in regular physical activity to maintain healthy lipid levels.

Pediatric hyperlipidemia is a condition where there are high levels of lipids in the blood in children. The condition can be caused by various factors, and early diagnosis and treatment are essential to prevent long-term complications such as cardiovascular disease. Treatment for hyperlipidemia involves lifestyle modifications and medication therapy, and prevention involves promoting healthy eating habits and physical activity from a young age.

CHAPTER 4

Neurology

Pediatric neurology is a medical specialty that deals with the diagnosis and treatment of disorders of the nervous system in children. Some of the common diagnoses that are treated by pediatric neurologists include:

1. Epilepsy: This is a neurological disorder that causes seizures, which can range from mild to severe.

2. Cerebral palsy: This is a group of disorders that affect movement and posture, and can be caused by brain damage during or shortly after birth.

3. Headaches: These are common complaints in children, and can be caused by a variety of conditions including migraines, tension headaches, or other neurological conditions.

4. Developmental delays: These are delays in reaching milestones such as sitting up, crawling, or walking, which can be caused by a variety of neurological disorders.

5. Attention deficit hyperactivity disorder (ADHD): This is a condition that affects attention, hyperactivity, and impulsivity, and can be caused by neurological factors.

6. Autism spectrum disorder (ASD): This is a developmental disorder that affects social interaction, communication, and behavior, and can have neurological causes.

7. Neuromuscular disorders: These are disorders that affect the nerves and muscles, such as muscular dystrophy or

spinal muscular atrophy.

8.   Tourette syndrome: This is a neurological disorder that causes repetitive, involuntary movements and vocalizations, called tics.

9.   Migraines: These are severe headaches that can be accompanied by other symptoms such as nausea, vomiting, or sensitivity to light and sound.

10. Stroke: Although less common in children than in adults, stroke can occur in children and can have neurological effects such as paralysis or speech difficulties.

Epilepsy

Pediatric epilepsy is a neurological condition that affects children and adolescents. It is characterized by seizures, which are abnormal electrical discharges in the brain that cause changes in behavior, movements, sensations, or consciousness. Epilepsy can be caused by a variety of factors, including genetic mutations, brain injury, infections, or metabolic disorders. In this discussion, we will cover the causes, symptoms, diagnosis, treatment, and management of pediatric epilepsy.

Causes of Epilepsy:

- Genetic factors: Some types of epilepsy are inherited, such as Dravet syndrome, Lennox-Gastaut syndrome, or Juvenile Myoclonic Epilepsy.
- Brain injury: Traumatic brain injury, stroke, or brain tumors can cause epilepsy.
- Infections: Encephalitis, meningitis, or other infections that affect the brain can cause epilepsy.
- Metabolic disorders: Disorders that affect the body's ability to process nutrients and chemicals, such as phenylketonuria, can cause epilepsy.
- Developmental disorders: Children with developmental disorders, such as autism or cerebral palsy, are at a higher

risk of developing epilepsy.

Symptoms of Epilepsy:

- Seizures: Seizures can take many different forms, depending on the part of the brain affected. Some seizures cause jerking movements, while others cause staring spells or loss of consciousness.
- Aura: Some children with epilepsy may experience a warning sign or aura before a seizure, such as a strange smell, taste, or feeling.
- Changes in behavior: Children with epilepsy may experience changes in behavior, such as irritability, mood swings, or aggression.
- Cognitive problems: Epilepsy can affect a child's cognitive abilities, including memory, attention, and language skills.

Diagnosis of Epilepsy:

- Physical exam: A doctor may perform a physical exam to look for signs of neurological problems, such as weakness or tremors.
- Electroencephalogram (EEG): An EEG measures the electrical activity in the brain and can detect abnormal patterns that are characteristic of epilepsy.
- Imaging tests: Magnetic resonance imaging (MRI) or computed tomography (CT) scans can help identify structural abnormalities or brain lesions that may be causing seizures.
- Blood tests: Blood tests can help identify genetic mutations or metabolic disorders that may be causing seizures.

Treatment and Management of Epilepsy:

- Medication: Anti-seizure medication is often the first line of treatment for pediatric epilepsy. These medications can help reduce the frequency and severity of seizures.
- Dietary therapy: Some children with epilepsy may benefit from a ketogenic diet, which is high in fat and low in carbohydrates.
- Surgery: In some cases, surgery may be an option to remove brain lesions or tissue that is causing seizures.
- Supportive care: Children with epilepsy may benefit from supportive care, such as physical therapy, speech therapy, or counseling to address emotional and social issues.

Epilepsy is a neurological disorder that can have a significant impact on a child's development and quality of life. Early diagnosis and treatment are essential to help manage seizures and prevent long-term complications. It is important for parents and caregivers to work closely with their healthcare providers to develop a comprehensive treatment plan that addresses the child's specific needs and goals.

Cerebral Palsy

Cerebral palsy is a neurological disorder that affects muscle control, movement, and coordination in children. It is caused by damage to the developing brain, which can occur before, during, or shortly after birth. In this discussion, we will cover the causes, symptoms, diagnosis, treatment, and management of pediatric cerebral palsy.

Causes of Cerebral Palsy:

- Brain injury: Brain injury can occur before, during, or shortly after birth, and can be caused by factors such as oxygen deprivation, infections, or traumatic injuries.
- Prematurity: Premature birth is a risk factor for cerebral palsy, as the brain may not have fully developed before

birth.

- Genetic factors: Some cases of cerebral palsy are caused by genetic mutations that affect brain development.
- Maternal factors: Maternal infections, exposure to toxins, or other maternal health issues can increase the risk of cerebral palsy.

Symptoms of Cerebral Palsy:

- Abnormal muscle tone: Children with cerebral palsy may have stiff or floppy muscles, making movement difficult or awkward.
- Delayed motor development: Children with cerebral palsy may have delayed motor milestones, such as rolling over, sitting up, or walking.
- Abnormal posture: Children with cerebral palsy may have an abnormal posture, such as scoliosis or a curved spine.
- Spasticity: Spasticity is a type of muscle stiffness that can cause jerky movements or difficulty with fine motor skills.
- Cognitive and developmental problems: Some children with cerebral palsy may have cognitive or developmental problems, such as intellectual disability or learning difficulties.

Diagnosis of Cerebral Palsy:

- Physical exam: A doctor may perform a physical exam to look for signs of abnormal muscle tone, motor development, or posture.
- Imaging tests: Magnetic resonance imaging (MRI) or computed tomography (CT) scans can help identify brain abnormalities or lesions that may be causing cerebral palsy.
- Developmental assessment: A developmental assessment can help identify cognitive or developmental

problems.

Treatment and Management of Cerebral Palsy:

- Physical therapy: Physical therapy can help children with cerebral palsy improve their muscle strength, coordination, and range of motion.
- Occupational therapy: Occupational therapy can help children with cerebral palsy improve their fine motor skills, such as writing or using utensils.
- Speech therapy: Speech therapy can help children with cerebral palsy improve their communication skills, such as speaking or using assistive devices.
- Medications: Medications such as muscle relaxants or anti-spasticity drugs can help reduce muscle stiffness and improve mobility.
- Surgery: In some cases, surgery may be an option to improve muscle function, such as tendon lengthening or muscle transfer surgery.
- Assistive devices: Assistive devices such as braces, splints, or wheelchairs can help children with cerebral palsy improve their mobility and independence.

Cerebral palsy is a complex neurological disorder that can have a significant impact on a child's development and quality of life. Early diagnosis and intervention are crucial to help manage symptoms and improve outcomes. It is important for parents and caregivers to work closely with their healthcare providers to develop a comprehensive treatment plan that addresses the child's specific needs and goals.

Headaches

Headaches are a common complaint in children and adolescents. They can have a significant impact on a child's daily activities and quality of life. In this discussion, we will cover the causes, types, symptoms, diagnosis, treatment, and management of pediatric headaches.

Causes of Headaches:

- Tension headaches: Tension headaches are the most common type of headache in children and are often caused by stress, anxiety, or muscle tension.
- Migraines: Migraines are a type of headache that can cause severe pain, nausea, vomiting, and sensitivity to light and sound. They may be triggered by certain foods, lack of sleep, or hormonal changes.
- Sinus headaches: Sinus headaches are caused by inflammation or infection of the sinuses.
- Cluster headaches: Cluster headaches are a rare type of headache that can cause severe pain, typically on one side of the head.
- Other causes: Other causes of pediatric headaches may include head injuries, infections, or underlying medical conditions such as brain tumors.

Symptoms of Headaches:

- Pain or pressure in the head
- Sensitivity to light or sound
- Nausea or vomiting
- Dizziness or lightheadedness
- Muscle tension in the neck or shoulders
- Irritability or mood changes

Diagnosis of Headaches:

- Medical history: A doctor will ask about the child's medical history, including any previous headaches or medical conditions.
- Physical exam: A physical exam can help rule out other causes of headaches, such as sinus or ear infections.
- Neurological exam: A neurological exam can help identify any underlying neurological issues that may be

causing headaches.

- Imaging tests: Imaging tests such as magnetic resonance imaging (MRI) or computed tomography (CT) scans may be used to rule out underlying medical conditions such as brain tumors.

Treatment and Management of Headaches:

- Lifestyle changes: Lifestyle changes such as getting enough sleep, eating a healthy diet, and reducing stress can help prevent headaches.
- Medications: Over-the-counter pain relievers such as acetaminophen or ibuprofen can help relieve mild to moderate headaches. For more severe headaches, prescription medications such as triptans or anti-nausea medications may be prescribed.
- Biofeedback: Biofeedback is a technique that uses relaxation exercises to help reduce stress and tension in the body, which can help prevent headaches.
- Cognitive-behavioral therapy (CBT): CBT is a type of therapy that can help children and adolescents develop coping strategies to manage stress and anxiety, which can help prevent headaches.
- Complementary therapies: Complementary therapies such as acupuncture or massage therapy may also be helpful in managing headaches.

Headaches can have a significant impact on a child's quality of life. It is important for parents and caregivers to work closely with their healthcare providers to develop a comprehensive treatment plan that addresses the child's specific needs and goals. With proper diagnosis, treatment, and management, most children with headaches can lead healthy, active lives.

Attention Deficit Hyperactivity Disorder

Attention Deficit Hyperactivity Disorder (ADHD) is a neurodevelopmental disorder that is characterized by difficulty with attention, hyperactivity, and impulsivity. The exact cause of ADHD is not known, but it is believed to be related to a combination of genetic, neurological, and environmental factors.

The signs and symptoms of pediatric ADHD include:

- Difficulty paying attention or staying focused
- Difficulty following instructions
- Difficulty completing tasks
- Forgetfulness
- Fidgeting or squirming
- Difficulty sitting still
- Excessive talking
- Difficulty waiting their turn
- Interrupting others

To diagnose ADHD, a pediatrician will typically perform a physical examination and ask about the child's symptoms and developmental history. The pediatrician may also refer the child to a specialist such as a child psychologist or a child neurologist for further evaluation. The diagnosis of ADHD is often made based on the criteria set out in the Diagnostic and Statistical Manual of Mental Disorders (DSM-5).

The treatment for ADHD typically includes:

- Medications such as stimulants (e.g. Ritalin, Adderall) to improve attention and reduce hyperactivity and impulsivity
- Behavioral therapy to teach the child strategies to manage their symptoms
- Parenting strategies to help the child manage their

symptoms
- School-based interventions to help the child succeed in the classroom
- Collaboration between the family, pediatrician, and school staff to support the child

Prognosis for ADHD varies, but with proper treatment, many children are able to improve their attention, hyperactivity, and impulsivity. However, ADHD is a chronic condition and some symptoms may persist into adulthood. It's important to continue monitoring the child's progress and adjusting treatment as needed.

Autism Spectrum Disorder

Autism Spectrum Disorder (ASD) is a neurodevelopmental disorder characterized by difficulties with social interaction, communication, and repetitive behaviors. The exact cause of ASD is not known, but it is believed to be related to a combination of genetic and environmental factors.

The signs and symptoms of pediatric autism may vary widely and can include:

- Difficulty with social interactions
- Limited or absent verbal communication
- Repetitive behaviors, such as rocking or flapping
- Difficulty with nonverbal communication
- Difficulty with imaginative play
- Sensory sensitivities
- Unusual interest in certain objects
- Lack of interest in social interactions

To diagnose autism, a pediatrician will typically perform a developmental screening and evaluation, which may include a thorough physical examination, review of the child's medical history, and referral to a specialist such as a developmental pediatrician or a child psychologist for a comprehensive evaluation. The diagnosis is often made based on criteria set out in the Diagnostic and Statistical Manual of Mental Disorders (DSM-5)

The treatment for pediatric autism typically includes:

- Behavioral therapy, such as Applied Behavior Analysis (ABA)
- Speech and language therapy
- Occupational therapy
- Medications to address specific symptoms such as anxiety or hyperactivity
- Special education and support services

Prognosis for autism varies widely and depends on the individual child's needs and the interventions that are provided. However, early diagnosis and intervention can lead to significant improvements in social interaction, communication, and adaptive behaviors. It's important to seek a pediatrician's guidance to address any concerns or symptoms, and to work with a team of specialists to create an individualized treatment plan that addresses the child's specific needs.

Neuromuscular Disorders

Neuromuscular disorders are a group of conditions that affect the muscles and/or the nerves that control them in children. These disorders can have a significant impact on a child's ability to move, breathe, and participate in daily activities. In this discussion, we will cover the causes, types, symptoms, diagnosis, treatment, and management of pediatric neuromuscular disorders.

Causes of Neuromuscular Disorders:

- Genetic mutations: Many neuromuscular disorders are caused by genetic mutations that affect the development or function of the muscles or nerves.
- Autoimmune disorders: Some neuromuscular disorders may be caused by the immune system attacking the muscles or nerves.
- Infections: Certain infections, such as polio or West Nile virus, can cause neuromuscular disorders.
- Environmental factors: Exposure to certain toxins or chemicals may increase the risk of developing neuromuscular disorders.

Types of Neuromuscular Disorders:

- Muscular dystrophy: Muscular dystrophy is a group of genetic disorders that cause progressive muscle weakness and degeneration.
- Spinal muscular atrophy (SMA): SMA is a genetic disorder that affects the motor neurons in the spinal cord, leading to muscle weakness and atrophy.
- Charcot-Marie-Tooth disease (CMT): CMT is a genetic disorder that affects the nerves in the limbs, leading to muscle weakness and atrophy.
- Myasthenia gravis: Myasthenia gravis is an autoimmune disorder that causes muscle weakness and fatigue.
- Congenital myopathies: Congenital myopathies are a group of genetic disorders that affect the development and function of the muscles.

Symptoms of Neuromuscular Disorders:

- Muscle weakness or atrophy
- Delayed motor development

- Difficulty walking or standing
- Breathing difficulties
- Difficulty with fine motor skills such as writing or buttoning clothes
- Fatigue
- Joint contracture

Diagnosis of Neuromuscular Disorders:

- Medical history: A doctor will ask about the child's medical history, including any family history of neuromuscular disorders.
- Physical exam: A physical exam can help identify muscle weakness or atrophy and may also include testing reflexes and muscle tone.
- Electromyography (EMG): EMG is a test that measures the electrical activity in the muscles and can help identify neuromuscular disorders.
- Genetic testing: Genetic testing may be used to identify the specific genetic mutation that is causing a neuromuscular disorder.

Treatment and Management of Neuromuscular Disorders:

- Physical therapy: Physical therapy can help improve muscle strength and mobility, as well as prevent joint contractures.
- Occupational therapy: Occupational therapy can help children learn new ways to perform daily activities and improve fine motor skills.
- Medications: Medications such as corticosteroids or immunosuppressants may be used to manage symptoms of certain neuromuscular disorders.
- Respiratory support: Children with neuromuscular disorders that affect breathing may require respiratory support, such as a ventilator or non-invasive ventilation.
- Surgery: Surgery may be recommended in some cases,

such as to correct joint contractures or scoliosis.

Pediatric neuromuscular disorders can have a significant impact on a child's daily activities and quality of life. It is important for parents and caregivers to work closely with their healthcare providers to develop a comprehensive treatment plan that addresses the child's specific needs and goals. With proper diagnosis, treatment, and management, most children with neuromuscular disorders can lead healthy, active lives

Tourette Syndrome

Tourette syndrome is a neurodevelopmental disorder that is characterized by repetitive, involuntary movements and vocalizations called tics. These tics can be simple, such as eye blinking or throat clearing, or complex, such as jumping or repeating phrases. In this discussion, we will cover the causes, symptoms, diagnosis, treatment, and management of pediatric Tourette syndrome.

Causes of Tourette Syndrome:

- Genetics: Tourette syndrome is believed to be caused by genetic mutations or abnormalities that affect the development or function of the brain.
- Neurotransmitters: Neurotransmitters are chemicals in the brain that transmit signals between neurons. Abnormalities in neurotransmitter function, specifically dopamine, have been linked to Tourette syndrome.
- Environmental factors: Some environmental factors, such as prenatal exposure to toxins or infections, may increase the risk of developing Tourette syndrome.

Symptoms of Tourette Syndrome:

- Motor tics: These tics are involuntary movements of the body, such as eye blinking, shoulder shrugging, or facial grimacing.

- Vocal tics: These tics are involuntary vocalizations, such as throat clearing, coughing, or repeating words or phrases.
- Coprolalia: Coprolalia is a vocal tic that involves saying socially inappropriate or obscene words or phrases. This is a rare symptom of Tourette syndrome, but it is often the most well-known and misunderstood symptom.
- Obsessive-compulsive symptoms: Many children with Tourette syndrome also have obsessive-compulsive symptoms, such as repetitive behaviors or thoughts.

Diagnosis of Tourette Syndrome:

- Medical history: A doctor will ask about the child's medical history, including any family history of Tourette syndrome.
- Physical exam: A physical exam can help identify any motor or vocal tics.
- Diagnostic criteria: The Diagnostic and Statistical Manual of Mental Disorders (DSM-5) provides diagnostic criteria for Tourette syndrome.
- Psychological evaluation: A psychological evaluation can help identify any coexisting conditions, such as anxiety or depression.

Treatment and Management of Tourette Syndrome:

- Behavioral therapy: Behavioral therapy can help children with Tourette syndrome learn to manage their tics and reduce their frequency and severity.
- Medications: Medications such as antipsychotics or alpha agonists may be used to manage symptoms of Tourette syndrome.
- Deep brain stimulation: Deep brain stimulation is a surgical procedure that involves implanting electrodes in the brain to regulate abnormal brain activity. This is

a relatively new treatment for Tourette syndrome and is usually reserved for severe cases that do not respond to other treatments.

Tourette syndrome is a complex disorder that can have a significant impact on a child's daily activities and quality of life. It is important for parents and caregivers to work closely with their healthcare providers to develop a comprehensive treatment plan that addresses the child's specific needs and goals. With proper diagnosis, treatment, and management, most children with Tourette syndrome can lead healthy, active lives.

Migraines

Migraines in the pediatric population are a common neurological disorder in children that is characterized by recurrent headaches that can be debilitating and affect a child's daily activities. In this discussion, we will cover the causes, symptoms, diagnosis, treatment, and management of pediatric migraines.

Causes of Migraines:

- Genetics: Migraines tend to run in families, suggesting a genetic component to the disorder.
- Environmental factors: Environmental factors such as stress, changes in sleep patterns, or changes in weather can trigger migraines in some children.
- Neurotransmitters: Neurotransmitters, such as serotonin and dopamine, play a role in regulating pain and mood and are believed to contribute to migraines.

Symptoms of Migraines:

- Headaches: The hallmark symptom of migraines is a moderate to severe headache that can last from a few hours to several days. The pain is often described as throbbing or pulsing and is typically located on one side of the head.
- Nausea and vomiting: Many children with migraines also experience nausea and vomiting during an episode.
- Sensitivity to light and sound: Migraines can make children more sensitive to light and sound, and they may seek out dark, quiet places to alleviate their symptoms.
- Aura: Some children may experience an aura before a migraine episode, which can involve visual disturbances, such as flashing lights or blind spots, or other neurological symptoms, such as tingling or numbness in the face or hands.

Diagnosis of Migraines:

- Medical history: A doctor will ask about the child's medical history, including any family history of migraines.
- Physical exam: A physical exam can help identify any signs of underlying medical conditions that may be causing the headaches.
- Diagnostic criteria: The International Classification of Headache Disorders provides diagnostic criteria for migraines in children.
- Neurological testing: In some cases, a neurological exam or imaging tests may be necessary to rule out other underlying conditions.

Treatment and Management of Migraines:

- Lifestyle changes: Lifestyle changes such as regular sleep patterns, stress management, and avoiding triggers can help reduce the frequency and severity of migraines.
- Medications: Medications such as ibuprofen,

acetaminophen, or triptans can be used to treat migraines. In some cases, preventative medications such as beta-blockers or antidepressants may be used to reduce the frequency of migraines.

- Behavioral therapy: Behavioral therapy can help children learn to manage stress and anxiety and cope with migraines.

Migraines can have a significant impact on a child's daily activities and quality of life. It is important for parents and caregivers to work closely with their healthcare providers to develop a comprehensive treatment plan that addresses the child's specific needs and goals. With proper diagnosis, treatment, and management, most children with migraines can lead healthy, active lives.

Stroke

Pediatric stroke is a rare but serious condition that occurs when blood flow to the brain is disrupted, leading to damage or death of brain cells. In this discussion, we will cover the causes, symptoms, diagnosis, treatment, and management of pediatric stroke.

Causes of Stroke:

- Congenital heart defects: Children with certain congenital heart defects are at higher risk of developing stroke due to a higher risk of blood clots or brain bleeding.
- Sickle cell disease: Children with sickle cell disease are at increased risk of stroke due to the sickle-shaped red blood cells that can clog blood vessels in the brain.
- Trauma: Head injuries or trauma can lead to damage to blood vessels in the brain, leading to stroke.
- Infection: Certain infections, such as meningitis or encephalitis, can lead to inflammation and blockage of blood vessels in the brain.

Symptoms of Stroke:

- Seizures: Seizures are a common symptom of pediatric stroke and can occur before, during, or after the stroke.
- Weakness or paralysis: Stroke can cause weakness or paralysis on one side of the body.
- Difficulty speaking or understanding: Stroke can affect language and communication abilities.
- Headache: Headaches can be a symptom of pediatric stroke.
- Vision changes: Stroke can cause vision changes or blindness in one or both eyes.
- Behavioral changes: Stroke can cause changes in behavior, such as confusion, irritability, or lethargy.

Diagnosis of Stroke:

- Medical history and physical exam: A doctor will ask about the child's medical history and symptoms and perform a physical exam to look for signs of stroke.
- Imaging tests: Imaging tests such as CT or MRI scans can help confirm the diagnosis and identify the location and extent of the stroke.
- Blood tests: Blood tests can help identify any underlying medical conditions that may be contributing to the stroke.

Treatment and Management of Stroke:

- Medications: Medications such as blood thinners, anti-seizure medications, or antibiotics may be used to treat stroke and any underlying medical conditions.
- Surgery: Surgery may be necessary in some cases to remove blood clots or repair damaged blood vessels in the brain.
- Rehabilitation: Rehabilitation, such as physical therapy, occupational therapy, and speech therapy, can

help children regain function and improve quality of life after a stroke.

Stroke is a serious condition that requires prompt diagnosis and treatment. Parents and caregivers should be aware of the risk factors and symptoms of pediatric stroke and seek medical attention immediately if they suspect a stroke has occurred. With early intervention and ongoing management, many children with stroke can make significant recoveries and lead healthy, active lives.

CHAPTER 5

Hematology and Oncology

Pediatric hematology and oncology is a medical specialty that deals with the diagnosis and treatment of blood disorders and cancers in children. Some of the common diagnoses that are treated by pediatric hematologists and oncologists include:

1. Leukemia: This is a cancer of the blood and bone marrow that affects the production of white blood cells.
2. Lymphoma: This is a cancer of the lymphatic system, which is part of the immune system and helps to fight infections.
3. Brain tumors: These are tumors that occur in the brain and can cause a variety of neurological symptoms.
4. Hemophilia: This is a bleeding disorder that affects the ability of the blood to clot properly.
5. Sickle cell anemia: This is a genetic blood disorder that causes abnormal red blood cells, leading to anemia and other complications.
6. Thrombocytopenia: This is a disorder in which the body has a low number of platelets, which are important for blood clotting.
7. Hemolytic anemia: This is a disorder in which the body destroys red blood cells faster than it can produce them.
8. Immune thrombocytopenic purpura (ITP): This is a disorder in which the immune system attacks platelets,

leading to a low platelet count.

9.   Neuroblastoma: This is a cancer that develops in the nerve cells of the sympathetic nervous system, which controls functions such as heart rate and blood pressure.

10. Wilms tumor: This is a cancer that affects the kidneys and is most commonly found in young children.

Treatment for these and other pediatric hematology and oncology diagnoses often includes a combination of chemotherapy, radiation therapy, and other specialized therapies, depending on the specific condition and individual needs of the child.

Leukemia

Leukemia is a type of cancer that affects the blood and bone marrow, which is the spongy tissue inside bones where blood cells are produced. In this discussion, we will cover the causes, symptoms, diagnosis, treatment, and management of pediatric leukemia.

Causes of Leukemia: The exact causes of pediatric leukemia are not fully understood. However, certain factors can increase a child's risk of developing leukemia, including:

- Genetics: Certain genetic mutations or disorders, such as Down syndrome, can increase the risk of developing leukemia.
- Environmental factors: Exposure to radiation or certain chemicals may increase the risk of developing leukemia.
- Immune system disorders: Children with certain immune system disorders may have an increased risk of developing leukemia.

Symptoms of Leukemia: The symptoms of pediatric leukemia can vary depending on the type of leukemia and the stage of the disease. Common symptoms include:

- Fatigue or weakness
- Fever
- Frequent infections
- Easy bruising or bleeding
- Bone or joint pain
- Enlarged lymph nodes, liver, or spleen
- Loss of appetite or weight loss
- Headaches

Diagnosis of Leukemia:

- Physical exam and medical history: A doctor will perform a physical exam and ask about the child's medical history and symptoms.
- Blood tests: Blood tests can help detect abnormal blood cell counts or the presence of leukemia cells in the blood.
- Bone marrow biopsy: A small sample of bone marrow is removed and examined under a microscope to look for leukemia cells.
- Imaging tests: Imaging tests such as CT scans or X-rays may be used to look for signs of leukemia in other parts of the body.

Treatment and Management of Leukemia:

- Chemotherapy: Chemotherapy is the primary treatment for pediatric leukemia and involves the use of drugs to kill cancer cells.
- Radiation therapy: Radiation therapy may be used in certain cases to kill cancer cells.
- Stem cell transplant: A stem cell transplant involves replacing the child's bone marrow with healthy stem cells from a donor.
- Supportive care: Supportive care, such as medications to manage side effects and nutritional support, may also be part of the treatment plan.

Leukemia is a serious condition that requires prompt diagnosis and treatment. Parents and caregivers should be aware of the risk factors and symptoms of pediatric leukemia and seek medical attention if they suspect their child may have the disease. With early intervention and ongoing management, many children with leukemia can make significant recoveries and lead healthy, active lives.

Lymphoma

Pediatric lymphoma is a type of cancer that affects the lymphatic system, which is a part of the immune system that helps fight infections. In this discussion, we will cover the causes, symptoms, diagnosis, treatment, and management of pediatric lymphoma.

Causes of Lymphoma: The exact causes of pediatric lymphoma are not fully understood. However, certain factors can increase a child's risk of developing lymphoma, including:

- Genetics: Certain genetic mutations or disorders, such as Down syndrome, can increase the risk of developing lymphoma.
- Environmental factors: Exposure to radiation or certain chemicals may increase the risk of developing lymphoma.
- Immune system disorders: Children with certain immune system disorders may have an increased risk of developing lymphoma.

Symptoms of Lymphoma: The symptoms of pediatric lymphoma can vary depending on the type of lymphoma and the stage of the disease. Common symptoms include:

- Swollen lymph nodes, which may be painless
- Fever

- Night sweats
- Unexplained weight loss
- Fatigue or weakness
- Loss of appetite
- Itchy skin or rash

Diagnosis of Lymphoma:

- Physical exam and medical history: A doctor will perform a physical exam and ask about the child's medical history and symptoms.
- Blood tests: Blood tests can help detect abnormal blood cell counts or the presence of lymphoma cells in the blood.
- Imaging tests: Imaging tests such as CT scans or X-rays may be used to look for signs of lymphoma in other parts of the body.
- Biopsy: A small sample of tissue is removed and examined under a microscope to look for lymphoma cells.

Treatment and Management of Lymphoma:

- Chemotherapy: Chemotherapy is the primary treatment for pediatric lymphoma and involves the use of drugs to kill cancer cells.
- Radiation therapy: Radiation therapy may be used in certain cases to kill cancer cells.
- Immunotherapy: Immunotherapy is a treatment that helps the immune system fight cancer cells.
- Stem cell transplant: A stem cell transplant involves replacing the child's bone marrow with healthy stem cells from a donor.
- Supportive care: Supportive care, such as medications to manage side effects and nutritional support, may also be part of the treatment plan.

Lymphoma is a serious condition that requires prompt diagnosis and treatment. Parents and caregivers should be aware of the risk factors and symptoms of pediatric lymphoma and seek medical attention if they suspect their child may have the disease. With early intervention and ongoing management, many children with lymphoma can make significant recoveries and lead healthy, active lives.

Brain Tumors

Pediatric brain tumors are a type of cancer that starts in the brain or spinal cord of children. They can be either benign or malignant and can affect children of any age, although they are more common in younger children. In this discussion, we will cover the causes, symptoms, diagnosis, treatment, and management of pediatric brain tumors.

Causes of Brain Tumors: The exact causes of pediatric brain tumors are not fully understood, but certain factors can increase a child's risk of developing a brain tumor, including:

- Genetics: Some inherited conditions, such as neurofibromatosis or Li-Fraumeni syndrome, can increase the risk of developing brain tumors.
- Exposure to radiation: Children who have received radiation therapy to the head and neck area have a higher risk of developing brain tumors.
- Immune system disorders: Children with certain immune system disorders may have an increased risk of developing brain tumors.

Symptoms of Brain Tumors: The symptoms of pediatric brain tumors can vary depending on the location and size of the tumor. Common symptoms include:

- Headaches, especially in the morning or worsen over time
- Nausea or vomiting
- Seizures

- Weakness or numbness in the arms or legs
- Difficulty with coordination or balance
- Vision or hearing changes
- Behavioral or personality changes
- Fatigue or drowsiness

Diagnosis of Brain Tumors:

- Physical exam and medical history: A doctor will perform a physical exam and ask about the child's medical history and symptoms.
- Neurological exam: A neurological exam checks the child's reflexes, strength, coordination, and sensation.
- Imaging tests: Imaging tests such as CT scans or MRI may be used to look for the presence of a brain tumor.
- Biopsy: A small sample of tissue is removed and examined under a microscope to look for cancer cells.

Treatment and Management of Brain Tumors:

- Surgery: Surgery may be performed to remove as much of the tumor as possible.
- Radiation therapy: Radiation therapy may be used to kill remaining cancer cells after surgery or to shrink the tumor before surgery.
- Chemotherapy: Chemotherapy is the use of drugs to kill cancer cells and is often used in combination with surgery and radiation therapy.
- Targeted therapy: Targeted therapy is a type of treatment that targets specific molecules within cancer cells to block their growth.
- Supportive care: Supportive care, such as medications to manage side effects and nutritional support, may also be part of the treatment plan.

Brain tumors are a serious condition that requires prompt

diagnosis and treatment. Parents and caregivers should be aware of the risk factors and symptoms of pediatric brain tumors and seek medical attention if they suspect their child may have the disease. With early intervention and ongoing management, many children with brain tumors can make significant recoveries and lead healthy, active lives.

Hemophilia

Hemophilia is a rare inherited bleeding disorder that affects the blood's ability to clot. It is usually diagnosed during childhood and is more common in boys than girls. In this discussion, we will cover the causes, symptoms, diagnosis, treatment, and management of pediatric hemophilia.

Causes of Hemophilia: Pediatric hemophilia is caused by a deficiency in one of the clotting factors that help the blood to clot. There are two main types of hemophilia:

- Hemophilia A: This is caused by a deficiency in clotting factor VIII.
- Hemophilia B: This is caused by a deficiency in clotting factor IX.

Both types of hemophilia are inherited from the child's parents, and symptoms can range from mild to severe depending on the level of clotting factor in the child's blood.

Symptoms of Hemophilia: The symptoms of pediatric hemophilia can vary depending on the severity of the condition. Common symptoms include:

- Frequent nosebleeds
- Bruising easily
- Bleeding into the muscles and joints, which can cause pain, swelling, and stiffness
- Blood in the urine or stool
- Prolonged bleeding after injuries or surgery

- Spontaneous bleeding without an obvious cause

Diagnosis of Hemophilia:

- Blood tests: Blood tests can measure the levels of clotting factors in the child's blood and confirm a diagnosis of hemophilia.
- Genetic testing: Genetic testing can determine whether the child has inherited hemophilia from their parents.

Treatment and Management of Hemophilia:

- Replacement therapy: This involves giving the child a replacement clotting factor to help their blood clot normally. The replacement clotting factor can be given through a vein or under the skin.
- Desmopressin: This is a medication that can stimulate the release of clotting factor VIII in mild cases of hemophilia A.
- Management of bleeding: If a child with hemophilia experiences bleeding, treatment may include rest, ice, compression, and elevation of the affected area. In severe cases, bleeding may require hospitalization and infusion of clotting factors.
- Physical therapy: Physical therapy can help children with hemophilia to maintain mobility and prevent joint damage.
- Counseling: Counseling can help children and families cope with the emotional and psychological effects of living with hemophilia.

Hemophilia is a rare but serious condition that requires ongoing management and treatment to prevent complications. With early diagnosis and appropriate treatment, children with hemophilia can lead healthy, active lives. Parents and caregivers should be aware of the signs and symptoms of hemophilia and seek medical attention if they suspect their child may have the condition.

Sickle Cell Anemia

Sickle cell anemia is a genetic disorder that affects the production of hemoglobin, a protein in red blood cells that carries oxygen throughout the body. The condition is inherited from a child's parents and primarily affects people of African descent. In this discussion, we will cover the causes, symptoms, diagnosis, treatment, and management of pediatric sickle cell anemia.

Causes of Sickle Cell Anemia:

Sickle cell anemia is caused by a mutation in the gene that produces hemoglobin. Normally, hemoglobin carries oxygen through the blood vessels. In sickle cell anemia, the abnormal hemoglobin causes the red blood cells to become stiff and sticky, forming a crescent or sickle shape. These sickle-shaped cells can block blood flow, leading to pain, organ damage, and other complications.

Symptoms of Sickle Cell Anemia: The symptoms of sickle cell anemia can vary in severity from mild to severe. Common symptoms include:

- Episodes of pain: This is known as a sickle cell crisis and can be severe enough to require hospitalization.
- Anemia: Sickle cell anemia can cause fatigue, weakness, and shortness of breath.
- Jaundice: Sickle cell anemia can cause the skin and eyes to turn yellow.
- Frequent infections: Sickle cell anemia can make children more susceptible to infections.
- Delayed growth and development: Sickle cell anemia can affect growth and development in children.

Diagnosis of Sickle Cell Anemia:

- Newborn screening: Most states in the U.S. require newborns to be screened for sickle cell anemia.
- Blood tests: Blood tests can confirm a diagnosis of sickle cell anemia and determine the severity of the condition.
- Genetic testing: Genetic testing can determine whether the child has inherited sickle cell anemia from their parents.

Treatment and Management of Sickle Cell Anemia:

- Pain management: Pain during sickle cell crises can be managed with pain medication.
- Hydroxyurea: This medication can help reduce the frequency and severity of sickle cell crises.
- Blood transfusions: In severe cases, blood transfusions may be necessary to increase the number of normal red blood cells in the body.
- Antibiotics: Antibiotics may be prescribed to prevent infections.
- Bone marrow transplant: In some cases, a bone marrow transplant may be considered as a potential cure for sickle cell anemia.

In addition to medical treatment, parents and caregivers can take steps to help manage the condition, such as:

- Keeping children hydrated to prevent dehydration, which can trigger sickle cell crises.
- Encouraging regular exercise to improve blood flow and promote overall health.
- Providing emotional support to help children and families cope with the challenges of living with sickle cell anemia.

Sickle cell anemia is a complex condition that requires ongoing management and treatment to prevent complications. With appropriate medical care and lifestyle changes, children with sickle cell anemia can lead healthy, active lives.

Thrombocytopenia

Thrombocytopenia is a medical condition characterized by a low platelet count in children. Platelets are small cells in the blood that help in the process of blood clotting. Children with thrombocytopenia have an increased risk of bleeding and bruising, which can range from mild to life-threatening. In this discussion, we will cover the causes, symptoms, diagnosis, treatment, and management of pediatric thrombocytopenia.

Causes of Thrombocytopenia: Pediatric thrombocytopenia can be caused by a variety of factors, including:

- Idiopathic thrombocytopenic purpura (ITP): A condition in which the body's immune system attacks platelets, leading to a low platelet count.
- Viral infections: Viral infections such as Epstein-Barr virus (EBV) and cytomegalovirus (CMV) can cause temporary thrombocytopenia.
- Medications: Certain medications such as antibiotics, anticonvulsants, and chemotherapy drugs can cause thrombocytopenia as a side effect.
- Inherited disorders: Inherited disorders such as Fanconi anemia and Wiskott-Aldrich syndrome can cause thrombocytopenia.
- Nutritional deficiencies: Deficiencies in vitamin B12, folate, or iron can lead to thrombocytopenia.

Symptoms of Thrombocytopenia: The symptoms of thrombocytopenia can vary depending on the severity of the condition. Common symptoms include:

- Easy bruising
- Bleeding gums
- Nosebleeds

- Prolonged bleeding after injury or surgery
- Petechiae (small red or purple spots on the skin)

Diagnosis of Thrombocytopenia:

- Blood tests: Blood tests can confirm the diagnosis of thrombocytopenia and determine the platelet count and other blood cell counts.
- Bone marrow aspiration: In some cases, a bone marrow aspiration may be performed to determine the cause of thrombocytopenia.

Treatment and Management of Thrombocytopenia: The treatment of pediatric thrombocytopenia depends on the underlying cause and the severity of the condition. Treatment options may include:

- Medications: Corticosteroids and intravenous immunoglobulin (IVIG) can be used to increase platelet counts in children with ITP.
- Blood transfusions: In severe cases of thrombocytopenia, a blood transfusion may be necessary to increase platelet counts.
- Surgery: In some cases, surgery may be necessary to stop bleeding.
- Lifestyle changes: Children with thrombocytopenia should avoid activities that increase the risk of bleeding, such as contact sports.

In addition to medical treatment, parents and caregivers can take steps to help manage the condition, such as:

- Monitoring for signs of bleeding and bruising
- Providing emotional support to help children and families cope with the challenges of living with thrombocytopenia.

Thrombocytopenia is a medical condition that requires

ongoing management and treatment to prevent complications. With appropriate medical care and lifestyle changes, children with thrombocytopenia can lead healthy, active lives.

Hemolytic Anemia

Hemolytic anemia is a medical condition in which red blood cells are destroyed faster than they can be replaced, leading to a deficiency in the number of red blood cells in the body. Red blood cells are important because they carry oxygen from the lungs to the rest of the body. When there are not enough red blood cells, the body does not get enough oxygen, leading to symptoms such as fatigue, weakness, and shortness of breath. In this discussion, we will cover the causes, symptoms, diagnosis, treatment, and management of pediatric hemolytic anemia.

Causes of Hemolytic Anemia: There are several different causes of pediatric hemolytic anemia, including:

- Inherited disorders: Hemolytic anemia can be caused by inherited disorders such as sickle cell disease, thalassemia, and hereditary spherocytosis.
- Autoimmune disorders: In some cases, hemolytic anemia can be caused by autoimmune disorders such as lupus and rheumatoid arthritis, in which the body's immune system attacks its own red blood cells.
- Infections: Certain infections, such as malaria and some types of hepatitis, can cause hemolytic anemia.
- Medications: Certain medications, such as antibiotics and chemotherapy drugs, can cause hemolytic anemia as a side effect.
- Toxins: Exposure to certain toxins, such as lead or snake venom, can cause hemolytic anemia.

Symptoms of Hemolytic Anemia: The symptoms of hemolytic

anemia can vary depending on the severity of the condition. Common symptoms include:

- Fatigue
- Weakness
- Shortness of breath
- Pale skin
- Yellowing of the skin and eyes (jaundice)
- Rapid heartbeat
- Enlarged spleen

Diagnosis of Hemolytic Anemia:

- Blood tests: Blood tests can confirm the diagnosis of hemolytic anemia and determine the number of red blood cells, as well as other blood cell counts and levels of bilirubin and lactate dehydrogenase (LDH).
- Bone marrow biopsy: In some cases, a bone marrow biopsy may be performed to determine the underlying cause of hemolytic anemia.

Treatment and Management of Hemolytic Anemia: The treatment of pediatric hemolytic anemia depends on the underlying cause and the severity of the condition. Treatment options may include:

- Blood transfusions: In severe cases of hemolytic anemia, a blood transfusion may be necessary to replace the lost red blood cells.
- Medications: Medications such as corticosteroids and immunosuppressants can be used to treat autoimmune hemolytic anemia.
- Surgery: In some cases, surgery may be necessary to remove the spleen, which can contribute to the destruction of red blood cells.
- Lifestyle changes: Children with hemolytic anemia should avoid activities that increase the risk of complications, such as contact sports.

In addition to medical treatment, parents and caregivers can take steps to help manage the condition, such as:

- Providing a healthy diet rich in iron and other nutrients to help support the production of red blood cells.
- Monitoring for signs of complications such as infections or blood clots.
- Providing emotional support to help children and families cope with the challenges of living with hemolytic anemia.

Hemolytic anemia is a medical condition that requires ongoing management and treatment to prevent complications. With appropriate medical care and lifestyle changes, children with hemolytic anemia can lead healthy, active lives.

Immune Thrombocytopenic Purpura (ITP)

Immune thrombocytopenic purpura (ITP) is a medical condition that affects the blood's ability to clot. It is characterized by low levels of platelets, which are necessary for clotting, resulting in abnormal bleeding and bruising. In this discussion, we will cover the causes, symptoms, diagnosis, treatment, and management of pediatric ITP.

Causes of Immune Thrombocytopenic Purpura: The exact cause of pediatric ITP is not known. However, it is believed to be an autoimmune disorder in which the body's immune system attacks its own platelets, leading to their destruction. This can result in low platelet counts and an increased risk of bleeding.

Symptoms of Immune Thrombocytopenic Purpura:

- Unusual bruising or bleeding

- Small red or purple spots on the skin (petechiae)
- Heavy menstrual periods in adolescent girls
- Nosebleeds or bleeding gums
- Blood in urine or stool
- Fatigue
- Enlarged spleen

Diagnosis of Immune Thrombocytopenic Purpura:

- Blood tests: Blood tests can confirm the diagnosis of ITP by measuring the number of platelets in the blood and ruling out other possible causes of low platelet counts.
- Bone marrow biopsy: In some cases, a bone marrow biopsy may be performed to rule out other possible causes of low platelet counts.

Treatment and Management of Immune Thrombocytopenic Purpura: The treatment of ITP depends on the severity of the condition and the child's age. Treatment options may include:

- Observation: In mild cases of ITP, observation may be all that is needed as the condition may resolve on its own within a few weeks or months.
- Medications: Medications such as corticosteroids, intravenous immunoglobulin (IVIG), and rituximab can be used to increase platelet counts.
- Surgery: In rare cases, surgery to remove the spleen may be necessary to prevent platelet destruction.
- Lifestyle changes: Children with ITP should avoid activities that increase the risk of bleeding, such as contact sports.

In addition to medical treatment, parents and caregivers can take steps to help manage the condition, such as:

- Providing a healthy diet rich in nutrients to help support the immune system and promote healing.
- Monitoring for signs of bleeding or other complications.

- Providing emotional support to help children and families cope with the challenges of living with ITP.

Immune thrombocytopenic purpura is a medical condition that requires ongoing management and treatment to prevent complications. With appropriate medical care and lifestyle changes, children with ITP can lead healthy, active lives.

Neuroblastoma

Neuroblastoma is a type of cancer that develops in immature nerve cells in infants and children. It is the most common solid tumor in infants and accounts for about 7-10% of all childhood cancers. In this discussion, we will cover the causes, symptoms, diagnosis, treatment, and management of pediatric neuroblastoma.

Causes of Neuroblastoma: The exact cause of pediatric neuroblastoma is not known. However, it is believed to occur when normal nerve cells undergo genetic mutations that cause them to grow and divide abnormally, resulting in the formation of a tumor.

Symptoms of Pediatric Neuroblastoma:

The symptoms of neuroblastoma can vary depending on the location and size of the tumor. Common symptoms may include:

- Abdominal swelling or mass
- Loss of appetite or weight loss
- Pain or tenderness in the abdomen
- Difficulty breathing or chest pain
- Bone pain
- Fatigue or weakness
- High blood pressure
- Eye changes, such as drooping eyelids or unequal pupils
- In rare cases, a child may have paraneoplastic syndrome,

a group of symptoms that occur when the tumor releases hormones or other substances that affect the body's normal function.

Diagnosis of Neuroblastoma:

- Physical exam: A doctor may perform a physical exam to check for signs of a tumor, such as a mass or swelling.
- Imaging tests: Imaging tests such as ultrasound, X-ray, CT scan, MRI, or MIBG scan can be used to locate the tumor and determine its size and spread.
- Biopsy: A biopsy involves removing a small sample of the tumor tissue for examination under a microscope to confirm the diagnosis of neuroblastoma.

Treatment and Management of Neuroblastoma: The treatment of pediatric neuroblastoma depends on the severity of the condition and the child's age. Treatment options may include:

- Surgery: Surgery is often the first step in treating neuroblastoma and involves removing as much of the tumor as possible.
- Chemotherapy: Chemotherapy is a treatment that uses drugs to kill cancer cells and may be used before or after surgery.
- Radiation therapy: Radiation therapy uses high-energy X-rays or other radiation to kill cancer cells and may be used after surgery or as a primary treatment.
- Immunotherapy: Immunotherapy is a newer treatment that uses the body's own immune system to target and kill cancer cells.
- High-dose chemotherapy with stem cell transplant: In some cases, a child may receive high-dose chemotherapy followed by a stem cell transplant to replace damaged cells.

In addition to medical treatment, parents and caregivers can take steps to help manage the condition, such as:

- Providing emotional support to help children and families cope with the challenges of living with neuroblastoma.
- Following a healthy diet to help support the immune system and promote healing.
- Monitoring for signs of recurrence or other complications.

Neuroblastoma is a serious condition that requires prompt diagnosis and treatment. With appropriate medical care and support, many children with neuroblastoma can recover and go on to lead healthy, active lives.

Wilm's Tumor

Wilms' tumor, also known as nephroblastoma, is a rare kidney cancer that mainly affects children under the age of 5. In this discussion, we will cover the causes, symptoms, diagnosis, treatment, and management of pediatric Wilms' tumor.

Causes of Wilms' Tumor: The exact cause of Wilms' tumor is not known. However, it is believed to occur when normal cells in the kidney undergo genetic mutations that cause them to grow and divide abnormally, resulting in the formation of a tumor. Certain genetic syndromes, such as Beckwith-Wiedemann syndrome and WAGR syndrome, can also increase the risk of developing Wilms' tumor.

Symptoms of Wilms' Tumor: The symptoms of Wilms' tumor can vary depending on the location and size of the tumor. Common symptoms may include:

- Abdominal swelling or mass
- Abdominal pain
- Loss of appetite or weight loss
- Blood in the urine
- High blood pressure

- Fever
- Nausea or vomiting
- Shortness of breath or difficulty breathing

Diagnosis of Wilms' Tumor:

- Physical exam: A doctor may perform a physical exam to check for signs of a tumor, such as a mass or swelling in the abdomen.
- Imaging tests: Imaging tests such as ultrasound, X-ray, CT scan, or MRI can be used to locate the tumor and determine its size and spread.
- Biopsy: A biopsy involves removing a small sample of the tumor tissue for examination under a microscope to confirm the diagnosis of Wilms' tumor.

Treatment and Management of Wilms' Tumor: The treatment of Wilms' tumor depends on the severity of the condition and the child's age. Treatment options may include:

- Surgery: Surgery is often the first step in treating Wilms' tumor and involves removing as much of the tumor as possible.
- Chemotherapy: Chemotherapy is a treatment that uses drugs to kill cancer cells and may be used before or after surgery.
- Radiation therapy: Radiation therapy uses high-energy X-rays or other radiation to kill cancer cells and may be used after surgery or as a primary treatment.
- Nephrectomy: If the tumor is large or has spread to other parts of the body, a nephrectomy may be necessary. This involves removing the affected kidney and surrounding tissues.

In addition to medical treatment, parents and caregivers can take steps to help manage the condition, such as:

- Providing emotional support to help children and

families cope with the challenges of living with Wilms' tumor.

- Following a healthy diet to help support the immune system and promote healing.
- Monitoring for signs of recurrence or other complications.

Wilms' tumor is a serious condition that requires prompt diagnosis and treatment. With appropriate medical care and support, many children with Wilms' tumor can recover and go on to lead healthy, active lives.

CHAPTER 6

Pulmonology

Pediatric pulmonology is a medical specialty that deals with the diagnosis and treatment of respiratory disorders in children. Some of the common diagnoses that are treated by pediatric pulmonologists include:

1. Asthma: This is a chronic condition that causes inflammation and narrowing of the airways, leading to wheezing, coughing, and shortness of breath.
2. Cystic fibrosis: This is a genetic disorder that affects the lungs, pancreas, and other organs, leading to thick, sticky mucus that can clog the airways and cause respiratory problems.
3. Bronchitis: This is an inflammation of the bronchial tubes, which carry air to and from the lungs, and can cause coughing and difficulty breathing.
4. Bronchiolitis
5. Pneumonia: This is an infection of the lungs that can be caused by bacteria, viruses, or other pathogens.
6. Sleep apnea: This is a condition in which breathing is disrupted during sleep, leading to snoring, gasping, or choking.
7. Congenital lung abnormalities: These are structural abnormalities of the lungs that are present at birth, such as lung hypoplasia or pulmonary sequestration.
8. Chronic cough: This is a persistent cough that lasts for

more than four weeks and can be caused by a variety of respiratory conditions.

9.   Respiratory distress syndrome: This is a condition that occurs in premature infants and causes difficulty breathing due to underdeveloped lungs.

10. Interstitial lung disease: This is a group of disorders that cause scarring and inflammation of the lung tissue, leading to breathing difficulties.

11. Tracheomalacia: This is a condition in which the cartilage in the trachea is weak or soft, causing the airway to collapse during breathing.

Treatment for these and other pediatric pulmonology diagnoses often includes a combination of medications, respiratory therapy, and other specialized interventions, depending on the specific condition and individual needs of the child.

Asthma

Asthma is a chronic respiratory disease that affects the airways, which carry air to and from the lungs. In asthma, the airways become inflamed and swollen, making it difficult to breathe. The inflammation and swelling can be triggered by a variety of environmental and lifestyle factors, including allergies, exercise, air pollution, and stress. Asthma affects people of all ages, but it often begins in childhood and is the most common chronic disease among children.

Symptoms of Asthma: The symptoms of asthma can vary in severity and frequency. Common symptoms include:

1.   Wheezing: A high-pitched whistling sound when breathing.

2.   Coughing: A persistent cough, especially at night or early in the morning.

3.   Shortness of breath: Difficulty breathing, especially

during physical activity.

4. Chest tightness: A feeling of tightness or pressure in the chest.

Triggers of Asthma: Asthma can be triggered by a variety of factors, including:

1. Allergens: Substances such as pollen, dust mites, animal dander, and mold.
2. Irritants: Substances such as tobacco smoke, air pollution, and strong odors.
3. Exercise: Physical activity can trigger asthma symptoms in some people.
4. Infections: Respiratory infections, such as the common cold or flu, can trigger asthma symptoms.
5. Stress: Emotional stress can trigger asthma symptoms in some people.

Diagnosis of Asthma: Asthma is diagnosed based on a combination of medical history, physical exam, and diagnostic tests. Common diagnostic tests include:

1. Spirometry: A lung function test that measures how much air you can inhale and exhale, and how quickly.
2. Peak flow measurement: A simple test that measures how quickly you can exhale air.
3. Chest X-ray: A radiographic image of the chest to rule out other respiratory conditions.
4. Allergy testing: Skin or blood tests to identify specific allergens that may be triggering asthma symptoms.

Treatment of Asthma: There is no cure for asthma, but it can be managed effectively with proper treatment. Treatment of asthma includes:

1. Medications: There are two main types of medications used to treat asthma: long-term control medications and quick-relief medications. Long-term control medications

are used daily to prevent asthma symptoms, while quick-relief medications are used as needed to treat sudden symptoms.

2. Inhalers: Inhalers are the most common way to deliver asthma medications. They work by delivering medication directly to the lungs.

3. Allergen avoidance: Avoiding exposure to allergens that trigger asthma symptoms is an important part of asthma management.

4. Asthma action plan: An asthma action plan is a written plan that outlines the steps to take if asthma symptoms worsen.

5. Asthma education: Asthma education is an important part of asthma management. It involves learning about asthma triggers, medications, and how to use inhalers properly.

Asthma is a chronic respiratory disease that affects the airways, making it difficult to breathe. Asthma can be triggered by a variety of environmental and lifestyle factors, and is diagnosed based on a combination of medical history, physical exam, and diagnostic tests. Treatment of asthma includes medications, inhalers, allergen avoidance, an asthma action plan, and asthma education. With proper management, people with asthma can live normal, active lives.

Cystic Fibrosis

Cystic fibrosis (CF) is a genetic disorder that affects the lungs, pancreas, and other organs. It is caused by mutations in the cystic fibrosis transmembrane conductance regulator (CFTR) gene, which results in the production of a defective protein that affects the transport of salt and water in and out of cells. This leads to the buildup of thick, sticky mucus in the lungs, pancreas, and other organs, causing a range of symptoms and complications.

Symptoms of Cystic Fibrosis: The symptoms of cystic fibrosis can vary in severity and may include:

1.   Respiratory symptoms: Chronic cough, wheezing, shortness of breath, frequent lung infections, and the production of thick, sticky mucus.
2.   Digestive symptoms: Poor growth and weight gain, frequent greasy, foul-smelling stools, abdominal pain, and bloating.
3.   Other symptoms: Salty-tasting skin, infertility in males, and sinus infections.

Complications of Cystic Fibrosis: Cystic fibrosis can lead to a number of complications, including:

1.   Respiratory complications: Chronic lung infections, bronchiectasis, and respiratory failure.
2.   Digestive complications: Pancreatic insufficiency, malnutrition, and diabetes.
3.   Other complications: Infertility, sinus infections, and liver disease.

Diagnosis of Cystic Fibrosis: Cystic fibrosis is diagnosed through a combination of medical history, physical exam, and diagnostic tests, including:

1.   Newborn screening: Many states in the United States require newborn screening for cystic fibrosis.
2.   Sweat test: The sweat test measures the amount of salt in sweat, which is usually elevated in people with cystic fibrosis.
3.   Genetic testing: Genetic testing can identify mutations in the CFTR gene that are associated with cystic fibrosis.
4.   Lung function tests: These tests measure lung capacity and how well the lungs are functioning.

Treatment of Cystic Fibrosis: There is no cure for cystic

fibrosis, but treatment can help manage symptoms and prevent complications. Treatment of cystic fibrosis includes:

1. Medications: Medications can help loosen and clear mucus from the lungs, prevent and treat infections, and improve digestion.
2. Airway clearance techniques: These techniques include chest physical therapy and breathing exercises that help clear mucus from the lungs.
3. Nutritional therapy: A high-calorie, high-protein diet and enzyme supplements can help improve digestion and promote growth and weight gain.
4. Lung transplant: In severe cases, a lung transplant may be necessary.

Cystic fibrosis is a genetic disorder that affects the lungs, pancreas, and other organs. It is caused by mutations in the CFTR gene, which results in the production of a defective protein that affects the transport of salt and water in and out of cells. Treatment of cystic fibrosis includes medications, airway clearance techniques, nutritional therapy, and, in severe cases, a lung transplant. With proper management, people with cystic fibrosis can live longer and healthier lives.

Bronchitis

Bronchitis is a common respiratory illness in children, characterized by inflammation and swelling of the bronchial tubes that carry air to and from the lungs. It can be caused by a viral or bacterial infection and often occurs after a cold or flu. Here is a detailed discussion of pediatric bronchitis.

Types of Bronchitis: There are two types of pediatric bronchitis:

1. Acute bronchitis: This is a short-term illness that usually lasts for a few weeks and is caused by a viral infection. It

can also be caused by exposure to irritants such as smoke or pollution.

2. Chronic bronchitis: This is a long-term illness that lasts for several months and is caused by exposure to irritants such as smoke or pollution. Chronic bronchitis is more common in adults than children.

Symptoms of Bronchitis: The symptoms of pediatric bronchitis may include:

1. Coughing: A persistent cough that lasts for several weeks is a common symptom of bronchitis. The cough may produce mucus or phlegm.
2. Wheezing: Wheezing is a high-pitched whistling sound that occurs when breathing.
3. Shortness of breath: Breathing may become difficult and shortness of breath may occur.
4. Chest discomfort: Pain or discomfort in the chest may occur.
5. Fatigue: A child may feel tired or weak due to the illness.

Diagnosis of Bronchitis: Pediatric bronchitis is diagnosed through a combination of medical history, physical exam, and diagnostic tests, including:

1. Physical exam: A doctor will listen to the child's chest with a stethoscope to check for wheezing, crackling or other abnormal sounds.
2. Medical history: The doctor will ask about the child's symptoms, medical history, and exposure to irritants such as smoke or pollution.
3. Chest X-ray: A chest X-ray can help identify any lung infections or other conditions that may be causing the symptoms.
4. Pulmonary function tests: These tests measure lung function and can help diagnose asthma or other respiratory conditions.

Treatment of Bronchitis: The treatment of pediatric bronchitis depends on the type and severity of the illness. Treatment options may include:

1. Rest and hydration: Rest and hydration can help the body fight off the infection and relieve symptoms.
2. Medications: Medications such as bronchodilators, antibiotics, and cough suppressants may be prescribed by a doctor to help treat symptoms and prevent complications.
3. Breathing treatments: Breathing treatments such as nebulizers or inhalers can help open up the airways and improve breathing.
4. Avoiding irritants: Avoiding irritants such as smoke or pollution can help prevent the condition from worsening.

Bronchitis is a common respiratory illness in children that is usually caused by a viral infection. Symptoms may include coughing, wheezing, shortness of breath, chest discomfort, and fatigue. Treatment options may include rest and hydration, medications, breathing treatments, and avoiding irritants. With proper management, pediatric bronchitis can be effectively treated and complications can be prevented.

Bronchiolitis

Bronchiolitis is a common respiratory illness in infants and young children that is characterized by inflammation of the bronchioles, which are the small airways in the lungs. It is most commonly caused by a viral infection, particularly respiratory syncytial virus (RSV), and usually occurs during the winter months. Here is a detailed discussion of pediatric bronchiolitis.

Symptoms of Bronchiolitis: The symptoms of pediatric bronchiolitis may include:

1. Coughing: A dry, hacking cough is a common symptom of bronchiolitis.
2. Wheezing: Wheezing is a high-pitched whistling sound that occurs when breathing.
3. Rapid breathing: Breathing may become rapid or shallow, and the child may use their abdominal muscles to help breathe.
4. Shortness of breath: Breathing may become difficult and shortness of breath may occur.
5. Fatigue: A child may feel tired or weak due to the illness.
6. Fever: A low-grade fever is common with bronchiolitis, but high fever is rare.
7. Decreased appetite: A child may have a decreased appetite and may not want to drink fluids.

Diagnosis of Bronchiolitis: Pediatric bronchiolitis is diagnosed through a combination of medical history, physical exam, and diagnostic tests, including:

1. Physical exam: A doctor will listen to the child's chest with a stethoscope to check for wheezing, crackling or other abnormal sounds.
2. Medical history: The doctor will ask about the child's symptoms, medical history, and exposure to other sick people or crowded places.
3. Chest X-ray: A chest X-ray can help identify any lung infections or other conditions that may be causing the symptoms.
4. Blood tests: Blood tests may be performed to check for signs of infection.
5. Nasal swab: A nasal swab can be used to test for RSV or other viral infections.

Treatment of Bronchiolitis: The treatment of pediatric bronchiolitis depends on the severity of the illness. Treatment options may include:

1. Rest and hydration: Rest and hydration can help the body fight off the infection and relieve symptoms.
2. Medications: Medications such as bronchodilators, steroids, and antivirals may be prescribed by a doctor to help treat symptoms and prevent complications.
3. Oxygen therapy: Oxygen therapy may be necessary if a child is having difficulty breathing.
4. Breathing treatments: Breathing treatments such as nebulizers or inhalers can help open up the airways and improve breathing.
5. Hospitalization: Hospitalization may be necessary for severe cases of bronchiolitis, particularly for infants under six months of age or those with other medical conditions.

Prevention of Bronchiolitis: Prevention measures for pediatric bronchiolitis include:

1. Handwashing: Frequent handwashing can help prevent the spread of viruses that cause bronchiolitis.
2. Vaccination: The RSV vaccine is currently not available, but the flu vaccine can help prevent some cases of bronchiolitis.
3. Avoiding exposure: Avoiding crowded places or people who are sick can help prevent the spread of viruses that cause bronchiolitis.

Bronchiolitis is a common respiratory illness in infants and young children that is usually caused by a viral infection, particularly RSV. Symptoms may include coughing, wheezing, rapid breathing, shortness of breath, fatigue, fever, and decreased appetite. Treatment options may include rest and hydration, medications, oxygen therapy, breathing treatments, and hospitalization for severe cases. Prevention measures include handwashing, vaccination, and avoiding exposure to sick individuals.

Pneumonia

Pneumonia is a lung infection that affects children and is caused by bacteria, viruses, or other microorganisms. It is a common condition that can be serious, especially in infants and young children. Here is a detailed discussion of pediatric pneumonia.

Causes of Pneumonia: Pediatric pneumonia can be caused by a variety of microorganisms, including:

1. Bacteria: Streptococcus pneumoniae, Haemophilus influenzae, and Mycoplasma pneumoniae are some of the most common bacterial causes of pneumonia in children.
2. Viruses: Respiratory syncytial virus (RSV), influenza virus, adenovirus, and parainfluenza virus are some of the most common viral causes of pneumonia in children.
3. Fungi: Fungal infections such as histoplasmosis and coccidioidomycosis can also cause pneumonia in children, although these are less common.

Symptoms of Pneumonia: The symptoms of pediatric pneumonia may vary depending on the cause, severity, and age of the child. Common symptoms may include:

1. Cough: A cough that produces phlegm or mucus is common with pneumonia.
2. Rapid breathing: Breathing may become rapid or shallow, and the child may use their abdominal muscles to help breathe.
3. Shortness of breath: Breathing may become difficult, and shortness of breath may occur.
4. Fever: A high fever is common with pneumonia,

although it may not always be present.

5.   Chest pain: Chest pain may occur, particularly when breathing deeply or coughing.

6.   Fatigue: A child may feel tired or weak due to the illness.

7.   Decreased appetite: A child may have a decreased appetite and may not want to eat or drink fluids.

Diagnosis of Pneumonia: Pediatric pneumonia is diagnosed through a combination of medical history, physical exam, and diagnostic tests, including:

1.   Physical exam: A doctor will listen to the child's chest with a stethoscope to check for crackling, wheezing or other abnormal sounds.

2.   Medical history: The doctor will ask about the child's symptoms, medical history, and exposure to other sick people or crowded places.

3.   Chest X-ray: A chest X-ray can help identify any lung infections or other conditions that may be causing the symptoms.

4.   Blood tests: Blood tests may be performed to check for signs of infection.

5.   Sputum culture: A sample of sputum (mucus coughed up from the lungs) can be tested for the presence of bacteria or other microorganisms.

Treatment of Pneumonia: The treatment of pneumonia depends on the cause and severity of the illness. Treatment options may include:

1.   Antibiotics: Antibiotics are often prescribed for bacterial pneumonia, and the specific antibiotic will depend on the type of bacteria causing the infection.

2.   Antiviral medications: Antiviral medications may be prescribed for viral pneumonia.

3.   Oxygen therapy: Oxygen therapy may be necessary if a child is having difficulty breathing.

4. Breathing treatments: Breathing treatments such as nebulizers or inhalers can help open up the airways and improve breathing.
5. Hospitalization: Hospitalization may be necessary for severe cases of pneumonia, particularly for infants under six months of age or those with other medical conditions.

Prevention of Pneumonia: Prevention measures for pediatric pneumonia include:

1. Vaccination: Vaccines are available for some of the common bacterial and viral causes of pneumonia, including the pneumococcal vaccine and the flu vaccine.
2. Handwashing: Frequent handwashing can help prevent the spread of germs that cause pneumonia.
3. Avoiding exposure: Avoiding exposure to tobacco smoke and other pollutants can also help reduce the risk of developing pneumonia.
4. Breastfeeding: Breastfeeding can help protect infants from infections, including pneumonia.
5. Proper hygiene: Encouraging proper hygiene, such as covering the mouth and nose when coughing or sneezing, can help prevent the spread of infection.
6. Good nutrition: A healthy diet can help support the immune system and reduce the risk of infection.

Complications of pneumonia can include:

1. Respiratory failure: In severe cases, pneumonia can cause respiratory failure, which can be life-threatening.
2. Pleural effusion: Pneumonia can cause fluid to accumulate in the space around the lungs, known as a pleural effusion.
3. Sepsis: Pneumonia can lead to sepsis, a potentially life-threatening condition in which the body's response to infection can cause damage to organs and tissues.
4. Lung abscess: A lung abscess can form when an area of

lung tissue becomes infected and forms a pocket of pus.

Pneumonia is a common condition that can be serious, especially in infants and young children. It can be caused by bacteria, viruses, or other microorganisms and is diagnosed through a combination of medical history, physical exam, and diagnostic tests. Treatment options depend on the cause and severity of the illness and may include antibiotics, antiviral medications, oxygen therapy, breathing treatments, and hospitalization. Prevention measures include vaccination, handwashing, avoiding exposure to pollutants, breastfeeding, proper hygiene, and good nutrition. Complications can include respiratory failure, pleural effusion, sepsis, and lung abscess.

Sleep Apnea

Sleep apnea is a condition where a child's breathing repeatedly stops and starts during sleep. It is caused by a blockage in the airway, which can be due to enlarged tonsils, adenoids, or other structural abnormalities in the throat or nose. This disruption in breathing can lead to decreased oxygen levels in the body, which can cause a variety of health problems. In this article, we will discuss pediatric sleep apnea in detail.

Symptoms: The most common symptoms of sleep apnea include:

1. Loud snoring
2. Pauses in breathing during sleep
3. Gasping or choking during sleep
4. Restless sleep or difficulty staying asleep
5. Excessive daytime sleepiness
6. Behavioral problems, such as hyperactivity and irritability
7. Poor academic performance
8. Headaches
9. Mouth breathing

10. Bedwetting

Causes: Sleep apnea is often caused by anatomical abnormalities, such as enlarged tonsils or adenoids, or structural problems in the nose or throat. Other risk factors include:

1. Obesity: Children who are overweight or obese are more likely to develop sleep apnea.
2. Family history: Sleep apnea can run in families.
3. Premature birth: Children who were born prematurely are at increased risk of developing sleep apnea.
4. Chronic nasal congestion: Chronic nasal congestion can lead to airway obstruction during sleep.
5. Medical conditions: Certain medical conditions, such as Down syndrome or cerebral palsy, can increase the risk of sleep apnea.

Diagnosis: Diagnosing sleep apnea involves a combination of medical history, physical exam, and diagnostic tests. The doctor will ask about the child's symptoms, medical history, and family history, and will perform a physical exam to look for signs of airway obstruction. Diagnostic tests may include:

1. Sleep study: A sleep study, or polysomnogram, is the most accurate way to diagnose sleep apnea. This test measures the child's breathing, heart rate, oxygen levels, and other factors during sleep.
2. X-ray or CT scan: Imaging tests may be done to look for structural abnormalities in the nose, throat, or airway.
3. Blood tests: Blood tests may be done to check for underlying medical conditions that could be causing sleep apnea.

Treatment: The treatment for sleep apnea depends on the severity of the condition and the underlying cause. Treatment options may include:

1.   Adenotonsillectomy: The most common treatment for sleep apnea in children is the removal of the tonsils and adenoids. This surgery can be very effective in relieving symptoms in children with mild to moderate sleep apnea.

2.   Continuous positive airway pressure (CPAP): CPAP is a machine that delivers a constant stream of air through a mask to keep the airway open during sleep. CPAP is often used in children with severe sleep apnea who are not good candidates for surgery.

3.   Oral appliances: Oral appliances, such as a mandibular advancement device, can help keep the airway open during sleep by moving the jaw forward.

4.   Weight loss: Children who are overweight or obese may benefit from weight loss, which can help reduce the severity of sleep apnea.

5.   Medications: Medications are generally not used to treat sleep apnea in children, but may be used in certain cases to relieve symptoms or to treat underlying medical conditions.

Sleep apnea is a common condition that can have serious health consequences if left untreated. It is caused by a blockage in the airway during sleep and can be diagnosed through a combination of medical history, physical exam, and diagnostic tests. Treatment options depend on the severity of the condition and the underlying cause, but may include surgery, CPAP, oral appliances, weight loss, and medication. It is important for parents and caregivers to be aware of the symptoms of sleep apnea and to seek medical attention if they suspect their child may be affected.

Untreated sleep apnea in children can lead to a range of health problems, including high blood pressure, heart disease, and behavioral problems. Children with sleep apnea may also be at increased risk of accidents and injuries due to daytime sleepiness. By seeking treatment for pediatric sleep apnea, parents can help their child sleep better, feel more rested, and improve their overall health and well-being.

Congenital Lung Abnormalities

Congenital lung abnormalities refer to structural abnormalities of the lungs that are present at birth. These abnormalities can affect the development and function of the lungs and can lead to respiratory problems in infants and children. In this article, we will discuss some of the most common congenital lung abnormalities in detail.

1. Pulmonary sequestration: Pulmonary sequestration is a rare congenital lung abnormality in which there is an abnormal blood supply to the lung tissue. This can cause the affected area of the lung to become non-functional and can lead to recurrent lung infections or respiratory distress. Treatment for pulmonary sequestration typically involves surgical removal of the affected lung tissue.

2. Congenital cystic adenomatoid malformation (CCAM): CCAM is a congenital lung abnormality in which there is overgrowth of lung tissue that forms cysts. This can lead to compression of healthy lung tissue and can cause respiratory distress, recurrent infections, and pneumothorax. Treatment for CCAM may involve surgery to remove the affected lung tissue.

3. Bronchogenic cysts: Bronchogenic cysts are rare congenital lung abnormalities that arise from the tracheobronchial tree. These cysts can cause compression of healthy lung tissue and can lead to recurrent infections and respiratory distress. Treatment for bronchogenic cysts typically involves surgical removal of the cysts.

4. Congenital lobar emphysema (CLE): CLE is a rare congenital lung abnormality in which there is overinflation of one or more lobes of the lung. This

can lead to compression of healthy lung tissue and can cause respiratory distress, recurrent infections, and pneumothorax. Treatment for CLE may involve surgery to remove the affected lung tissue.

5.   Tracheal stenosis: Tracheal stenosis is a congenital lung abnormality in which the trachea is abnormally narrow or obstructed. This can cause respiratory distress and may require surgical correction to relieve the obstruction and improve breathing.

6.   Pulmonary hypoplasia: Pulmonary hypoplasia is a congenital lung abnormality in which the lungs are underdeveloped or smaller than normal. This can cause respiratory distress and can lead to complications such as pulmonary hypertension and heart failure. Treatment for pulmonary hypoplasia may involve supportive measures such as oxygen therapy and mechanical ventilation.

7.   Congenital diaphragmatic hernia (CDH): CDH is a congenital lung abnormality in which there is a defect in the diaphragm that allows abdominal organs to move into the chest cavity. This can lead to compression of healthy lung tissue and can cause respiratory distress and other complications. Treatment for CDH typically involves surgery to repair the diaphragmatic defect and reposition the abdominal organs.

Congenital lung abnormalities are structural abnormalities of the lungs that are present at birth. These abnormalities can lead to respiratory problems in infants and children and may require surgical or supportive treatment. It is important for parents and caregivers to be aware of the signs and symptoms of congenital lung abnormalities and to seek medical attention if they suspect their child may be affected.

Chronic Cough

Chronic cough is defined as a cough that persists for more

than 4 weeks in children. It is a common problem in pediatric patients and can be caused by a variety of underlying conditions. In this article, we will discuss some of the most common causes of pediatric chronic cough in detail.

1. Asthma: Asthma is a chronic respiratory condition that causes inflammation and narrowing of the airways, leading to wheezing, shortness of breath, and coughing. In children, asthma is a common cause of chronic cough. Treatment for asthma typically involves the use of inhaled bronchodilators and corticosteroids to reduce inflammation and improve airway function.

2. Gastroesophageal reflux disease (GERD): GERD is a condition in which stomach acid flows back into the esophagus, causing irritation and inflammation. In children, GERD can cause chronic cough, as well as symptoms such as heartburn and regurgitation. Treatment for GERD may involve lifestyle changes, such as avoiding certain foods and eating smaller, more frequent meals, as well as the use of medication to reduce stomach acid production.

3. Postnasal drip: Postnasal drip occurs when excess mucus drips down the back of the throat, causing irritation and coughing. It is a common cause of chronic cough in children, especially during cold and allergy season. Treatment for postnasal drip may involve the use of nasal sprays, antihistamines, and decongestants to reduce congestion and mucus production.

4. Chronic bronchitis: Chronic bronchitis is a type of chronic obstructive pulmonary disease (COPD) that causes inflammation and narrowing of the bronchial tubes, leading to coughing and difficulty breathing. In children, chronic bronchitis may be caused by exposure to environmental irritants such as cigarette smoke or air pollution. Treatment for chronic bronchitis may involve the use of bronchodilators and corticosteroids to reduce

inflammation and improve airway function.

5.   Cystic fibrosis: Cystic fibrosis is a genetic disorder that affects the lungs, digestive system, and other organs. It causes the production of thick, sticky mucus that clogs the airways, leading to chronic coughing and respiratory infections. Treatment for cystic fibrosis typically involves a combination of airway clearance techniques, inhaled medications, and antibiotics to prevent and treat infections.

Chronic cough is a common problem in children that can be caused by a variety of underlying conditions. It is important for parents and caregivers to seek medical attention if their child has a persistent cough, as early diagnosis and treatment can help improve outcomes and prevent complications. Treatment for pediatric chronic cough will depend on the underlying cause and may involve lifestyle changes, medication, and other therapies.

Respiratory Distress Syndrome

Respiratory distress syndrome (RDS) is a common respiratory disorder that occurs in premature infants, typically those born before 34 weeks gestation. It is caused by a deficiency of surfactant, a substance that helps to keep the air sacs in the lungs open and prevent them from collapsing. In this article, we will discuss the pathophysiology, clinical presentation, diagnosis, and treatment of RDS in the pediatric population in detail.

Pathophysiology: Surfactant deficiency results in decreased lung compliance, which leads to a decreased functional residual capacity (FRC) and increased work of breathing. The resulting hypoxemia, hypercapnia, and acidosis can lead to respiratory failure if left untreated.

Clinical presentation: Infants with RDS may present with

tachypnea, grunting, nasal flaring, chest retractions, and cyanosis. They may also have low oxygen saturation levels and an increased carbon dioxide level in the blood. In severe cases, infants may require mechanical ventilation to support their breathing.

Diagnosis: Diagnosis of RDS is based on clinical presentation and confirmed by chest x-ray findings of diffuse bilateral pulmonary opacities with air bronchograms. Arterial blood gas analysis can help assess the severity of the respiratory failure.

Treatment:The primary treatment for RDS is surfactant replacement therapy, which can be given via endotracheal tube. The goal of therapy is to improve lung function, decrease the need for mechanical ventilation, and reduce the risk of complications such as pneumothorax and chronic lung disease. The use of nasal continuous positive airway pressure (CPAP) or high flow nasal cannula (HFNC) can also be used to provide respiratory support in less severe cases.

Other supportive measures include maintaining a neutral thermal environment, avoiding excessive handling and stimulation, and providing adequate nutrition and hydration. In severe cases, infants may require mechanical ventilation with positive end-expiratory pressure (PEEP) to support their breathing.

Prevention:Prevention of RDS involves the use of antenatal corticosteroids, which can help to accelerate lung maturity in preterm infants. Delivery of preterm infants in a tertiary care center with neonatal intensive care unit (NICU) capabilities can also help to improve outcomes.

Respiratory distress syndrome is a common respiratory disorder that occurs in premature infants due to surfactant deficiency. It is important to recognize the clinical signs and symptoms of RDS, as prompt diagnosis and treatment can improve outcomes and reduce the risk of complications. Surfactant replacement therapy is the mainstay of treatment, and prevention involves the use of antenatal corticosteroids and delivery in a tertiary care center with NICU capabilities.

Interstitial Lung Disease

Pediatric interstitial lung disease (ILD) is a group of rare disorders that affect the lung tissue and air sacs (alveoli) and can cause chronic respiratory failure. In this article, we will discuss the pathophysiology, clinical presentation, diagnosis, and treatment of pediatric ILD in detail.

Pathophysiology: ILD in children can be caused by a variety of factors, including genetic disorders, autoimmune diseases, and exposure to environmental toxins. These conditions can lead to inflammation and scarring of the lung tissue, which can result in decreased lung function and oxygenation.

Clinical presentation: The clinical presentation of pediatric ILD can vary depending on the underlying cause of the disease. Infants and young children may present with failure to thrive, tachypnea, and recurrent respiratory infections. Older children may present with cough, dyspnea, and exercise intolerance. In severe cases, children may require oxygen therapy and mechanical ventilation to support their breathing.

Diagnosis: Diagnosis of ILD involves a thorough evaluation of the patient's medical history, physical examination, and laboratory and imaging studies. Laboratory tests may include pulmonary function tests, arterial blood gas analysis, and genetic testing. Imaging studies, such as chest X-rays and high-resolution computed tomography (HRCT), can help to identify abnormalities in lung structure and function. In some cases, lung biopsy may be required to confirm the diagnosis.

Treatment: The treatment of ILD depends on the underlying cause of the disease. In some cases, supportive care such as oxygen therapy and respiratory support may be necessary. Corticosteroids and other immunosuppressive agents may be used to reduce inflammation and slow the progression of the disease in children with autoimmune-related ILD. Other treatments, such as antibiotics or antifungal medications, may be necessary to treat underlying infections.

In some cases, lung transplantation may be considered for children with end-stage disease. It is important for children with ILD to receive ongoing monitoring and management of their disease to prevent complications and optimize their lung function.

Prevention: Prevention of ILD involves avoiding exposure to environmental toxins and promoting healthy behaviors such as good nutrition and exercise. Genetic counseling may also be recommended for families with a history of inherited ILD.

Interstitial lung disease is a rare group of disorders that can cause chronic respiratory failure. Early recognition and diagnosis of the disease are essential to provide appropriate treatment and prevent complications. Treatment of pediatric ILD depends on the underlying cause of the disease and may include supportive care, immunosuppressive medications, and lung transplantation. Prevention of ILD involves avoiding exposure to environmental toxins and promoting healthy behaviors.

Tracheomalacia

Tracheomalacia is a rare condition characterized by a weakened or floppy trachea, which can cause breathing difficulties in children. In this article, we will discuss the pathophysiology, clinical presentation, diagnosis, and treatment of pediatric tracheomalacia in detail.

Pathophysiology: The trachea is a tube-like structure that carries air from the nose and mouth to the lungs. In children with tracheomalacia, the walls of the trachea are weak and cannot support the airway as it should, leading to narrowing or collapse of the trachea during inspiration or expiration. This can cause breathing difficulties, particularly during exercise or feeding.

Clinical presentation: The clinical presentation of tracheomalacia can vary depending on the severity of the condition. Infants and young children may present with noisy breathing (stridor), difficulty feeding, choking, or coughing. Older children may present with shortness of breath, chest pain, or exercise intolerance. In severe cases, children may require oxygen therapy and mechanical ventilation to support their breathing.

Diagnosis: Diagnosis of tracheomalacia involves a thorough evaluation of the patient's medical history, physical examination, and imaging studies. A flexible bronchoscopy, which is a procedure that allows direct visualization of the trachea and bronchi, is often used to confirm the diagnosis. Additional tests may include pulmonary function tests, CT scan, or MRI.

Treatment: The treatment of tracheomalacia depends on the severity of the condition. In mild cases, close observation may be sufficient. In more severe cases, treatment may include medication, surgery, or the use of a mechanical breathing support device.

Medication: Medications may be used to reduce inflammation and improve breathing. Bronchodilators, steroids, or other anti-inflammatory medications may be prescribed to help manage symptoms.

Surgery: Surgery may be recommended in cases where the tracheomalacia is severe and causing significant breathing difficulties. Tracheostomy, which involves creating an opening in the trachea through the neck, may be recommended in some cases. In other cases, a procedure known as tracheal stenting may be used to support the weakened trachea.

Mechanical breathing support: In some cases, a mechanical breathing support device such as a continuous positive airway pressure (CPAP) machine or a bi-level positive airway pressure (BiPAP) machine may be used to support breathing.

Tracheomalacia is a rare condition that can cause breathing difficulties in children. Diagnosis of tracheomalacia involves a thorough evaluation of the patient's medical history, physical examination, and imaging studies. Treatment may include medication, surgery, or the use of a mechanical breathing support device. It is important for children with tracheomalacia to receive ongoing monitoring and management of their condition to prevent complications and optimize their breathing.

CHAPTER 7

Rheumatology

Pediatric rheumatology is a medical specialty that deals with the diagnosis and treatment of autoimmune and inflammatory disorders in children. Some of the common diagnoses that are treated by pediatric rheumatologists include:

1. Juvenile idiopathic arthritis (JIA): This is the most common type of arthritis in children, characterized by joint pain, swelling, and stiffness.
2. Systemic lupus erythematosus (SLE): This is an autoimmune disease that can affect multiple organs, including the skin, kidneys, and joints.
3. Dermatomyositis: This is an inflammatory disease that affects the muscles and skin, causing muscle weakness and skin rashes.
4. Scleroderma: This is a rare autoimmune disease that causes hardening and thickening of the skin and internal organs.
5. Kawasaki disease: This is an acute illness that affects the blood vessels, causing fever, rash, and other symptoms.
6. Systemic onset juvenile rheumatoid arthritis: This is a subtype of JIA that also involves systemic symptoms, such as fever and rash.
7. Reactive arthritis: This is a type of arthritis that develops after an infection, such as a bacterial or viral infection.

8. Vasculitis: This is a group of disorders that cause inflammation and damage to the blood vessels, leading to a variety of symptoms depending on the affected organs.
9. Henoch-Schönlein purpura: This is a type of vasculitis that affects the small blood vessels, causing a rash and joint pain.
10. Behçet's disease: This is a rare autoimmune disease that causes inflammation of the blood vessels and can affect multiple organs, including the eyes, skin, and joints.

Treatment for these and other pediatric rheumatology diagnoses often includes a combination of medications, physical therapy, and other specialized interventions, depending on the specific condition and individual needs of the child.

Juvenile Idiopathic Arthritis

Juvenile Idiopathic Arthritis (JIA) is a type of arthritis that affects children under the age of 16 years old. JIA is a chronic disease that can cause joint inflammation, pain, stiffness, and swelling, and can result in long-term disability if left untreated.

There are several types of JIA, each with its own set of symptoms and characteristics. The most common types of JIA are oligoarticular, polyarticular, and systemic.

Oligoarticular JIA is the most common type of JIA and usually affects only a few joints, typically in the knees, ankles, or wrists. Polyarticular JIA affects multiple joints and can be further divided into two subtypes: rheumatoid factor-positive and rheumatoid factor-negative. Systemic JIA, also known as Still's disease, affects the whole body, causing fever, rash, and other symptoms in addition to joint pain and inflammation.

The exact cause of JIA is not known, but it is thought to be an autoimmune disease, where the immune system mistakenly attacks the body's own tissues, including the joints. Genetics, environmental factors, and infections may also play a role in the development of JIA.

Treatment for JIA focuses on reducing inflammation, relieving pain, and preserving joint function. This may include a combination of medications, physical therapy, and occupational therapy. In some cases, surgery may be necessary to repair or replace damaged joints.

The prognosis for children with JIA varies depending on the type and severity of the disease, but with proper treatment, many children are able to lead normal, active lives. It is important for children with JIA to receive ongoing medical care and monitoring to manage their symptoms and prevent long-term complications.

Systemic Lupus Erythematosus (SLE)

Systemic Lupus Erythematosus (SLE) is a chronic autoimmune disease that can affect multiple organs and systems in the body, including the skin, joints, kidneys, lungs, and nervous system. It is a rare disease that primarily affects children under the age of 18.

The exact cause of SLE is unknown, but it is thought to be a combination of genetic and environmental factors. The disease is more common in girls than boys, and certain ethnic groups, such as African Americans, Hispanics, and Asians, are at higher risk.

Symptoms of SLE can vary widely and may include fatigue, joint pain and stiffness, skin rashes, fever, weight loss, and oral ulcers. In some cases, pSLE can also cause more serious complications, such as kidney damage, seizures, or inflammation of the heart or lungs.

Diagnosis of SLE involves a thorough medical evaluation, including a physical exam, blood tests, and imaging studies. Doctors may also perform a biopsy of affected tissue to confirm the diagnosis.

Treatment for SLE typically involves a combination of medications, including nonsteroidal anti-inflammatory drugs (NSAIDs) for pain and inflammation, corticosteroids to reduce inflammation and suppress the immune system, and immunosuppressive drugs to prevent the immune system from attacking healthy tissues. In some cases, additional medications may be prescribed to treat specific symptoms or complications.

Children with SLE should receive ongoing medical care and monitoring to manage their symptoms and prevent long-term complications. With proper treatment, many children with SLE are able to lead normal, active lives.

In addition to medical treatment, lifestyle modifications, such as eating a healthy diet, getting regular exercise, and avoiding triggers that may worsen symptoms, can also be helpful in managing SLE.

Systemic lupus erythematosus is a chronic disease that requires ongoing management, with proper treatment and care, many children with the condition are able to achieve a good quality of life.

Dermatomyositis (DM)

Dermatomyositis (DM) is a rare autoimmune disorder that primarily affects children under the age of 18. It is characterized by inflammation of the muscles and skin, which can lead to muscle weakness, skin rashes, and other symptoms.

The exact cause of DM is unknown, but it is thought to be a combination of genetic and environmental factors. The disease is more common in girls than boys, and certain ethnic groups, such as African Americans and Asians, are at higher risk.

Symptoms of DM can vary widely and may include muscle weakness, difficulty swallowing, skin rashes, joint pain and stiffness, fatigue, and fever. In some cases, pDM can also cause more serious complications, such as lung disease or inflammation of the heart or blood vessels.

Diagnosis of DM involves a thorough medical evaluation, including a physical exam, blood tests, imaging studies, and a muscle biopsy to confirm the diagnosis.

Treatment for DM typically involves a combination of medications, including corticosteroids to reduce inflammation and suppress the immune system, immunosuppressive drugs to prevent the immune system from attacking healthy tissues, and intravenous immunoglobulin (IVIG) to boost the immune system. Physical therapy and rehabilitation may also be recommended to help manage muscle weakness and maintain function.

Ongoing medical care and monitoring to manage their symptoms and prevent long-term complications. With proper treatment, many children with pDM are able to achieve a good quality of life.

In addition to medical treatment, lifestyle modifications, such as eating a healthy diet, getting regular exercise, and avoiding triggers that may worsen symptoms, can also be helpful in managing pDM.

Dermatomyositis is a chronic disease that requires ongoing management, with proper treatment and care, many children with the condition are able to achieve a good quality of life.

Scleroderma

Scleroderma, also known as juvenile systemic sclerosis, is a rare autoimmune disease that primarily affects children under the age of 18. It is characterized by excessive growth of connective tissue, which can lead to skin thickening, organ damage, and other symptoms.

The exact cause of scleroderma is unknown, but it is thought to be a combination of genetic and environmental factors. The disease is more common in girls than boys, and certain ethnic groups, such as African Americans and Native Americans, are at higher risk.

Symptoms of scleroderma can vary widely depending on the subtype of the disease. The two main subtypes are localized scleroderma and systemic sclerosis.

Localized scleroderma primarily affects the skin and typically presents with one or more oval-shaped patches of thickened skin. Systemic sclerosis, on the other hand, can affect multiple organs and systems in the body, including the skin, joints, and internal organs. Symptoms of systemic sclerosis may include skin thickening, joint pain and stiffness, muscle weakness, digestive problems, lung disease, and heart disease.

Diagnosis of scleroderma involves a thorough medical evaluation, including a physical exam, blood tests, imaging studies, and skin biopsy to confirm the diagnosis.

Treatment for scleroderma typically involves a combination of medications, including immunosuppressive drugs to prevent the immune system from attacking healthy tissues, and other medications to manage specific symptoms and complications. Physical therapy and rehabilitation may also be recommended to help manage muscle weakness and maintain function.

It is important for children with scleroderma to receive ongoing medical care and monitoring to manage their symptoms and prevent long-term complications. With proper treatment, many children with pediatric scleroderma are able to achieve a good quality of life.

In addition to medical treatment, lifestyle modifications, such as eating a healthy diet, getting regular exercise, and avoiding triggers that may worsen symptoms, can also be helpful in managing scleroderma.

Overall, while pediatric scleroderma is a chronic disease that requires ongoing management, with proper treatment and care, many children with the condition are able to achieve a good quality of life.

Kawasaki Disease

Kawasaki Disease (KD), also known as mucocutaneous lymph node syndrome, is a rare illness that primarily affects children under the age of 5. It is characterized by inflammation of blood vessels throughout the body, which can lead to a range of symptoms.

The exact cause of KD is unknown, but it is thought to be a combination of genetic and environmental factors. The disease is more common in boys than girls and is more prevalent in certain ethnic groups, such as Asians and Pacific Islanders.

Symptoms of KD typically develop in phases and can vary widely between patients. The early phase of the disease may include a high fever that lasts for at least five days, a rash, redness and swelling of the hands and feet, and redness of the eyes.

In the later phases of the disease, children may experience peeling skin on their hands and feet, joint pain, abdominal pain, vomiting, diarrhea, and swollen lymph nodes.

Diagnosis of KD involves a thorough medical evaluation, including a physical exam, blood tests, and an echocardiogram to evaluate the heart for any signs of damage.

Treatment for KD typically involves hospitalization and administration of high-dose intravenous immunoglobulin (IVIG) and aspirin to reduce inflammation and prevent blood clots. Children with more severe symptoms or complications may require additional treatments, such as corticosteroids, other immunosuppressive drugs, or surgery.

Children with KD require prompt medical treatment to prevent complications, such as coronary artery aneurysms, which can lead to long-term heart damage.

Kawasaki Disease is a serious illness that requires prompt treatment, the vast majority of children with the disease recover fully with appropriate care. With early diagnosis and proper treatment, most children with KD can achieve a good quality of life.

Systemic Onset Juvenile Rheumatoid Arthritis (SoJIA)

Pediatric systemic onset juvenile rheumatoid arthritis (SoJIA) is a type of juvenile idiopathic arthritis (JIA) that primarily affects children under the age of 16. It is characterized by inflammation in multiple joints and organs throughout the body, which can lead to a range of symptoms.

The exact cause of SoJIA is unknown, but it is thought to be a combination of genetic and environmental factors. The disease is more common in girls than boys and typically begins before the age of 5.

Symptoms of SoJIA typically include a high fever that lasts for at least two weeks, a rash, joint pain and swelling, and inflammation in internal organs such as the liver, spleen, and lymph nodes. Other symptoms may include fatigue, weight loss, and anemia.

Diagnosis of SoJIA involves a thorough medical evaluation, including a physical exam, blood tests, and imaging studies to evaluate the joints and internal organs.

Treatment for SoJIA typically involves a combination of medications, including nonsteroidal anti-inflammatory drugs (NSAIDs), disease-modifying antirheumatic drugs (DMARDs), and biologic agents, which target specific components of the immune system to reduce inflammation.

In addition to medication, physical therapy and rehabilitation may also be recommended to help maintain joint mobility and function.

Children with SoJIA should receive ongoing medical care and monitoring to manage their symptoms and prevent long-term complications, such as joint damage or organ failure.

Systemic Onset Juvenile Rheumatoid Arthritis is a chronic disease that requires ongoing management, with proper treatment and care, many children with the condition are able to achieve a good quality of life.

Reactive Arthritis

Reactive arthritis (ReA) is a type of arthritis that typically develops in response to an infection elsewhere in the body, such as in the gastrointestinal or urinary tract. It primarily affects children and adolescents and can cause inflammation in multiple joints, as well as other symptoms.

The exact cause of ReA is not fully understood, but it is thought to be an autoimmune reaction triggered by an infection. The disease is more common in boys than girls and typically develops after an infection.

Symptoms of ReA typically include joint pain and swelling, especially in the knees, ankles, and feet. Other symptoms may include eye inflammation, skin rash, and urinary symptoms such as pain or frequent urination.

Diagnosis of ReA involves a thorough medical evaluation, including a physical exam, blood tests, and imaging studies to evaluate the joints and internal organs. Tests may also be done to identify any underlying infections that may be contributing to the symptoms.

Treatment for ReA typically involves a combination of medications, including nonsteroidal anti-inflammatory drugs (NSAIDs) to reduce pain and inflammation, and antibiotics if there is an underlying infection. In some cases, corticosteroids or other immunosuppressive drugs may be recommended to control inflammation.

Physical therapy and rehabilitation may also be recommended to help maintain joint mobility and function.

Ongoing medical care and monitoring to manage their symptoms and prevent long-term complications, such as joint damage.

Reactive Arthritis is a chronic disease that requires ongoing management, with proper treatment and care, many children with the condition are able to achieve a good quality of life.

Vasculitis

Vasculitis is a group of rare autoimmune diseases that cause inflammation in blood vessels throughout the body. The inflammation can damage blood vessels, leading to a range of symptoms and complications.

There are several types of pediatric vasculitis, including Kawasaki disease, Henoch-Schonlein purpura (HSP), polyarteritis nodosa (PAN), and granulomatosis with polyangiitis (GPA), among others. The exact cause of these diseases is not fully understood, but they are thought to be caused by a combination of genetic and environmental factors.

Symptoms of vasculitis can vary widely depending on the type of vasculitis and which organs are affected. Common symptoms include fever, joint pain and swelling, skin rash or lesions, abdominal pain, and organ dysfunction such as kidney or lung problems.

Diagnosis of vasculitis involves a thorough medical evaluation, including a physical exam, blood tests, and imaging studies to evaluate the blood vessels and organs. In some cases, a biopsy may be necessary to confirm the diagnosis.

Treatment for vasculitis typically involves a combination of medications, including corticosteroids, immunosuppressive drugs, and biologic agents, which target specific components of the immune system to reduce inflammation.

In addition to medication, physical therapy and rehabilitation may also be recommended to help maintain joint mobility and function, as well as to manage any long-term complications.

Children with vasculitis need to receive ongoing medical care and monitoring to manage their symptoms and prevent long-term complications, such as organ damage.

Although vasculitis is a chronic disease that requires ongoing management, with proper treatment and care, many children with the condition are able to achieve a good quality of life. Early diagnosis and treatment are key to preventing long-term complications and improving outcomes for children with vasculitis.

Henoch-Schönlein purpura (HSP)

Henoch-Schönlein purpura (HSP) is a type of vasculitis, which is an inflammation of the blood vessels. It is a rare condition that primarily affects children between the ages of 2 and 11. HSP is characterized by a rash of purple-red spots on the skin, joint pain and swelling, and gastrointestinal symptoms.

The exact cause of HSP is not known, but it is thought to be an autoimmune reaction triggered by an infection or other environmental factor. HSP is not contagious and cannot be spread from person to person.

Symptoms of HSP typically include a rash of purple-red spots on the skin, usually on the legs and buttocks, joint pain and swelling, abdominal pain, and sometimes bloody stools. In severe cases, HSP can also cause kidney damage, leading to protein in the urine, high blood pressure, and kidney failure.

Diagnosis of HSP involves a thorough medical evaluation, including a physical exam, blood tests, and sometimes a biopsy of the skin or kidney tissue to confirm the diagnosis.

Treatment for HSP typically involves management of symptoms, such as pain relief and anti-inflammatory medications, as well as bed rest and hydration for more severe cases. In some cases, corticosteroids or other immunosuppressive drugs may be recommended to control inflammation and prevent long-term complications, such as kidney damage.

Most cases of HSP resolve on their own within a few

weeks, and children generally make a full recovery. However, in some cases, HSP can cause long-term complications, particularly if there is kidney involvement. It is important for children with HSP to receive ongoing medical care and monitoring to manage their symptoms and prevent long-term complications.

Henoch-Schönlein purpura is a rare condition, with proper treatment and care, most children with the condition are able to achieve a full recovery and go on to lead healthy, normal lives.

Behcet's Disease

Behcet's disease is a rare autoimmune disorder that affects blood vessels throughout the body, leading to inflammation and damage to various organs and tissues. The condition primarily affects children and young adults, with onset usually occurring between the ages of 10 and 30.

The exact cause of Behcet's disease is not known, but it is thought to be an autoimmune disorder, in which the body's immune system mistakenly attacks its own tissues. Genetics and environmental factors may also play a role in the development of the condition.

Symptoms of Behcet's disease can vary widely, depending on which organs and tissues are affected. Common symptoms include mouth sores, genital sores, skin lesions, joint pain and swelling, eye inflammation, and central nervous system symptoms such as headaches and confusion.

Diagnosis of Behcet's disease involves a thorough medical evaluation, including a physical exam, blood tests, and imaging studies to evaluate the blood vessels and organs. In some cases, a biopsy may be necessary to confirm the diagnosis.

Treatment for Behcet's disease typically involves a combination of medications, including corticosteroids, immunosuppressive drugs, and biologic agents, which target specific components of the immune system to reduce inflammation. In addition to medication, physical therapy and rehabilitation may also be recommended to help maintain joint mobility and function.

Children with disease will require ongoing medical care and monitoring to manage their symptoms and prevent long-term complications, such as organ damage. In some cases, the condition may go into remission and the child may experience long periods of symptom-free living.

While Behcet's disease is a chronic condition that requires ongoing management, with proper treatment and care, many children with the condition are able to achieve a good quality of life. Early diagnosis and treatment are key to preventing long-term complications and improving outcomes for children with Behcet's disease.

CHAPTER 8

Nephrology

Pediatric nephrology is a medical specialty that deals with the diagnosis and treatment of kidney disorders in children. Some of the common diagnoses that are treated by pediatric nephrologists include:

1. Nephrotic syndrome: This is a kidney disorder that causes protein to leak into the urine, leading to swelling, fluid retention, and other symptoms.
2. Glomerulonephritis: This is a group of kidney disorders that cause inflammation of the glomeruli, the tiny filters in the kidneys that remove waste and excess fluids from the blood.
3. Hemolytic uremic syndrome: This is a rare but serious condition that can cause kidney failure, anemia, and low platelet count.
4. Acute kidney injury: This is a sudden loss of kidney function that can be caused by a variety of factors, including dehydration, infections, and medications.
5. Chronic kidney disease: This is a progressive loss of kidney function that can lead to kidney failure over time.
6. Urinary tract infections: These are infections of the urinary tract, including the bladder, kidneys, and ureters, that can cause pain, fever, and other symptoms.
7. Congenital kidney abnormalities: These are structural abnormalities of the kidneys that are present at birth,

such as kidney dysplasia or obstructive uropathy.

8. Nephritis: This is a type of kidney inflammation that can be caused by infections, autoimmune disorders, and other factors.

9. Renal tubular acidosis: This is a condition in which the kidneys are unable to maintain the proper balance of acids and bases in the blood.

10. Kidney stones: These are hard, mineral deposits that can form in the kidneys and cause pain, urinary tract infections, and other complications.

Treatment for these and other pediatric nephrology diagnoses often includes a combination of medications, dietary changes, and other specialized interventions, depending on the specific condition and individual needs of the child. In some cases, children with kidney disorders may require dialysis or kidney transplantation.

Nephrotic Syndrome

Nephrotic syndrome is a kidney disorder that affects children, characterized by the excretion of a large amount of protein in the urine, resulting in edema (swelling) and other symptoms. It is the most common glomerular disorder in childhood and is usually diagnosed between the ages of 2 and 6 years.

The exact cause of nephrotic syndrome is not known, but it is thought to be related to an abnormal immune system response that causes damage to the glomeruli, which are tiny blood vessels in the kidneys that filter waste and excess fluid from the blood. Certain infections, medications, and genetic factors may also play a role in the development of the condition.

Symptoms of nephrotic syndrome include swelling in the legs, ankles, and feet, as well as the hands and face, due to fluid accumulation in the body. The child may also experience fatigue, decreased appetite, and weight gain due to fluid retention. The child may also experience foamy urine due to the high amount of protein excreted.

Diagnosis of nephrotic syndrome involves a series of tests, including urine tests to measure protein excretion, blood tests to assess kidney function, and sometimes a kidney biopsy to confirm the diagnosis and determine the underlying cause of the condition.

Treatment for nephrotic syndrome typically involves the use of corticosteroids, which reduce inflammation in the kidneys and decrease the amount of protein excreted in the urine. Other medications, such as immunosuppressive drugs or diuretics, may also be used in combination with corticosteroids to manage symptoms and reduce the risk of complications.

In addition to medication, lifestyle modifications, such as limiting salt intake and increasing fluid intake, may also be recommended to help manage symptoms and prevent complications. The child may also require regular monitoring of kidney function and protein levels in the urine to assess the effectiveness of treatment and adjust medications as needed.

Overall, while nephrotic syndrome is a chronic condition that requires ongoing management, with proper treatment and care, many children with the condition are able to achieve a good quality of life. Early diagnosis and treatment are key to preventing long-term complications and improving outcomes for children with nephrotic syndrome.

Glomerulonephritis

Glomerulonephritis is a group of kidney diseases that affect the glomeruli, which are tiny blood vessels in the kidneys that filter waste and excess fluid from the blood. The condition is more common in children than adults, and it can cause significant damage to the kidneys if left untreated.

The exact cause of glomerulonephritis is not known, but it is thought to be related to an abnormal immune system response that causes inflammation in the glomeruli, leading to damage and scarring of the kidneys. In some cases, the condition may be triggered by an infection or an autoimmune disorder.

Symptoms of glomerulonephritis vary depending on the specific type of the condition but often include hematuria (blood in the urine), proteinuria (excessive protein in the urine), hypertension, edema (swelling), and decreased urine output. Other symptoms may include fatigue, headache, and loss of appetite.

Diagnosis of glomerulonephritis involves a series of tests, including blood and urine tests to assess kidney function and identify any underlying infections or autoimmune disorders. A kidney biopsy may also be necessary to confirm the diagnosis and determine the type and severity of the condition.

Treatment for glomerulonephritis depends on the specific type and severity of the condition but often involves the use of corticosteroids and immunosuppressive drugs, which reduce inflammation and slow down the progression of the disease. Blood pressure medication may also be prescribed to control hypertension, and diuretics may be used to reduce swelling and fluid retention.

In addition to medication, lifestyle modifications, such as limiting salt intake and increasing fluid intake, may also be recommended to help manage symptoms and prevent complications. The child may also require regular monitoring of kidney function and protein levels in the urine to assess the effectiveness of treatment and adjust medications as needed.

Gomerulonephritis is a serious condition that can cause long-term kidney damage if left untreated, with proper diagnosis and treatment, many children with the condition are able to achieve a good quality of life. Early diagnosis and treatment are key to preventing long-term complications and improving outcomes for children with glomerulonephritis.

Hemolytic Uremic Syndrome

Hemolytic uremic syndrome (HUS) is a rare but serious kidney disorder that primarily affects children under the age of 5. It is characterized by the destruction of red blood cells, the formation of blood clots, and acute kidney failure. HUS is most commonly caused by a type of bacteria called Shiga toxin-producing Escherichia coli (STEC), which is commonly found in contaminated food or water.

Symptoms of HUS often begin with diarrhea, which may be bloody, and abdominal pain. Over time, the child may develop fever, vomiting, and decreased urine output, as well as signs of anemia, such as fatigue, pale skin, and shortness of breath. As the disease progresses, the child may develop edema (swelling) in the arms and legs, and may become confused or disoriented.

Diagnosis of HUS involves a series of tests, including blood and urine tests to assess kidney function and identify any underlying infections or disorders. A stool culture may also be necessary to identify the presence of STEC bacteria.

Treatment for HUS typically involves supportive care, including fluids and electrolyte replacement, to manage symptoms and prevent complications. The child may also require blood transfusions to treat anemia, and in some cases, dialysis may be necessary to support kidney function.

Antibiotics are not usually used to treat HUS, as they may actually increase the risk of complications. Instead, medications such as anticoagulants or plasma exchange may be used to reduce the risk of blood clots and improve kidney function.

Hemolytic Uremic Syndrome is a serious condition that can cause long-term kidney damage if left untreated, with proper diagnosis and treatment, many children with the condition are able to recover fully. Early diagnosis and prompt treatment are key to preventing long-term complications and improving outcomes for children with HUS.

Acute Kidney Injury

Acute kidney injury (AKI), also known as acute renal failure, is a sudden and often reversible decrease in kidney function, resulting in a build-up of waste products and excess fluid in the body. The condition can be caused by a variety of factors, including dehydration, medication toxicity, infections, and kidney damage from injury or trauma.

Symptoms of AKI may include decreased urine output, swelling in the legs or feet, nausea, vomiting, fatigue, and confusion. In severe cases, the condition can lead to life-threatening complications, such as seizures, coma, and respiratory failure.

Diagnosis of AKI involves a series of tests, including blood and urine tests to assess kidney function, as well as imaging tests, such as ultrasound or CT scans, to evaluate the kidneys and urinary tract for any structural abnormalities.

Treatment for AKI depends on the underlying cause and severity of the condition. In some cases, AKI may resolve on its own with supportive care, such as fluid and electrolyte replacement, and avoiding medications or substances that may be causing the kidney injury. However, in more severe cases, hospitalization may be necessary, and treatment may involve medications or procedures to improve kidney function or address any underlying infections or injuries.

In some cases, dialysis may be necessary to remove excess fluid and waste products from the body when the kidneys are no longer able to do so effectively. Dialysis may be temporary, until kidney function improves, or may be required long-term in cases of chronic kidney disease.

Acute kidney injury can be a serious condition, prompt diagnosis and treatment can often lead to a good prognosis. In some cases, however, AKI can lead to chronic kidney disease or permanent kidney damage, so it is important to seek medical attention if any symptoms of kidney injury are present. Maintaining good overall health and avoiding substances or medications that can damage the kidneys can also help prevent the development of AKI.

Chronic Kidney Disease

Pediatric chronic kidney disease (CKD) is a long-term condition in which the kidneys gradually lose function over time. It can affect children of all ages and can be caused by a variety of factors, including congenital anomalies of the kidneys, inherited genetic disorders, infections, autoimmune diseases, and medications.

Symptoms of CKD may be mild or absent in the early stages of the condition, but can progress over time to include fatigue, decreased appetite, weight loss, high blood pressure, anemia, bone pain, and difficulty concentrating. In advanced stages, CKD can lead to complications such as heart disease, bone disease, and nerve damage.

Diagnosis of CKD involves a series of tests, including blood and urine tests to assess kidney function, as well as imaging tests, such as ultrasound or CT scans, to evaluate the kidneys and urinary tract for any structural abnormalities.

Treatment for CKD aims to slow the progression of the disease and manage symptoms. In some cases, medications may be prescribed to lower blood pressure, treat anemia, or address underlying infections or autoimmune disorders. In more advanced cases, dialysis or kidney transplant may be necessary to replace kidney function and improve quality of life, and, in addition to medical treatment, children with CKD may benefit from lifestyle changes, such as following a kidney-friendly diet, staying hydrated, and avoiding substances that can further damage the kidneys, such as tobacco and alcohol.

Chronic Kidney Disease is a serious condition that requires ongoing medical management, with proper treatment and lifestyle modifications, many children with the condition are able to lead full and active lives. Regular monitoring and management of the condition are essential to prevent complications and ensure the best possible outcomes for children with CKD.

Urinary Tract Infections

Urinary tract infections (UTIs) are common infections that can affect any part of the urinary tract, including the kidneys, bladder, ureters, and urethra. UTIs are more common in females than males, and are caused by bacteria entering the urinary tract through the urethra.

Symptoms of a UTI may include frequent urination, pain or burning during urination, cloudy or strong-smelling urine, and lower abdominal pain. In more severe cases, a UTI can cause fever, chills, and back pain.

Diagnosis of a UTI typically involves a urine test to check for the presence of bacteria and white blood cells in the urine. In some cases, imaging tests, such as an ultrasound or CT scan, may be used to evaluate the urinary tract for any structural abnormalities.

Treatment for a UTI typically involves a course of antibiotics to eliminate the infection. In addition to antibiotics, over-the-counter pain relievers and home remedies, such as drinking plenty of water and avoiding irritants such as caffeine and alcohol, may be helpful in managing symptoms.

Prevention of UTIs involves maintaining good hygiene, such as wiping from front to back after using the bathroom, staying well-hydrated, and avoiding irritants that can cause urinary tract irritation or inflammation.

In some cases, recurrent UTIs may be a sign of an underlying condition, such as kidney stones or an abnormality in the urinary tract. In these cases, further evaluation and treatment may be necessary to prevent future UTIs and complications.

Urinary Tract Infections can be uncomfortable and inconvenient, with proper treatment and prevention strategies, most UTIs can be resolved without complications.

Congenital Kidney Abnormalities

Pediatric congenital kidney abnormalities refer to structural abnormalities of the kidneys that are present at birth. These abnormalities can range from minor anomalies that do not cause any significant problems, to severe abnormalities that can affect kidney function and require medical management.

Some examples of congenital kidney abnormalities in children include:

1.   Renal agenesis: This is a condition where one or both kidneys do not develop in the womb. Children

with unilateral renal agenesis usually have no significant symptoms, while those with bilateral renal agenesis often have significant kidney dysfunction and require medical management.

2. Duplex kidney: This is a condition where a child has two ureters that drain into a single kidney. Duplex kidney can increase the risk of UTIs and kidney stones, and may require medical management.

3. Polycystic kidney disease (PKD): This is a genetic disorder that causes cysts to form in the kidneys, leading to progressive kidney damage. PKD can be present in infants or children, and can cause hypertension, kidney stones, and kidney failure.

4. Hydronephrosis: This is a condition where urine accumulates in the kidney due to a blockage in the ureter or bladder. Hydronephrosis can be caused by a variety of factors, including congenital anomalies, and can cause kidney damage if left untreated.

5. Multicystic dysplastic kidney (MCDK): This is a condition where one kidney has multiple cysts and does not function properly. MCDK is usually asymptomatic and does not require medical management, but in severe cases, surgical intervention may be necessary.

Diagnosis of congenital kidney abnormalities in children typically involves imaging tests, such as ultrasound or CT scans, to evaluate the kidneys and urinary tract for any structural abnormalities. Treatment for these conditions depends on the severity of the abnormality and may involve medical management, surgical intervention, or close monitoring and observation.

Congenital kidney abnormalities can be a serious condition, with proper management and treatment, many children with these conditions are able to lead full and healthy lives. Early diagnosis and treatment are important to prevent complications and ensure the best possible outcomes for children with congenital kidney abnormalities.

Nephritis

Nephritis is a term used to describe inflammation of the kidneys in children. Nephritis can be caused by a variety of factors, including infections, autoimmune disorders, and medications.

Some common types of nephritis include:

1. Acute poststreptococcal glomerulonephritis (APSGN): This is a type of nephritis that occurs following a streptococcal infection, such as strep throat or impetigo. APSGN is most common in children between the ages of 6 and 10 years old and can cause symptoms such as fever, fatigue, and swelling of the face and body. Most cases of APSGN resolve on their own within a few weeks, but in some cases, medical management may be necessary.

2. Lupus nephritis: This is a type of nephritis that occurs in children with systemic lupus erythematosus (SLE), an autoimmune disorder. Lupus nephritis can cause a variety of symptoms, including swelling of the face and legs, high blood pressure, and blood in the urine. Treatment for lupus nephritis typically involves medications to manage the underlying autoimmune disorder and prevent further kidney damage.

3. IgA nephropathy: This is a type of nephritis that occurs when the kidneys are unable to properly filter a protein called IgA. IgA nephropathy can cause symptoms such as blood in the urine and swelling of the face and legs. Treatment for IgA nephropathy may involve medications to manage symptoms and prevent further kidney damage.

4. Minimal change disease: This is a type of nephritis that is most common in young children. Minimal change

disease is characterized by damage to the small blood vessels in the kidneys, which can cause protein to leak into the urine. Minimal change disease is often treated with medications that suppress the immune system.

Diagnosis of nephritis typically involves blood and urine tests to evaluate kidney function and look for signs of inflammation or infection. In some cases, a kidney biopsy may be necessary to determine the underlying cause of the nephritis.

Treatment for nephritis depends on the underlying cause and severity of the condition. In many cases, medications to manage symptoms and prevent further kidney damage may be necessary. In severe cases, dialysis or kidney transplant may be necessary.

Nephritis can be a serious condition, with proper diagnosis and treatment, many children with nephritis are able to manage their symptoms and prevent further kidney damage. Regular monitoring and follow-up with a pediatric nephrologist is important for children with nephritis to ensure the best possible outcomes.

Renal Tubular Acidosis

Pediatric renal tubular acidosis (RTA) is a condition that occurs when the kidneys are unable to properly maintain the body's acid-base balance, resulting in an accumulation of acid in the bloodstream. There are several types of RTA, each with its own underlying cause.

1. Type 1 RTA: This is the most common form of pediatric RTA and is caused by a defect in the kidney's ability to reabsorb bicarbonate, a key component of the body's acid-base balance. Children with type 1 RTA may experience symptoms such as frequent urination, dehydration, and fatigue. Treatment for type 1 RTA typically involves

oral supplements of bicarbonate and potassium to help restore the body's acid-base balance.

2.   Type 2 RTA: This form of RTA is caused by a defect in the kidney's ability to reabsorb both bicarbonate and sodium. Children with type 2 RTA may experience symptoms such as weakness, fatigue, and dehydration. Treatment for type 2 RTA typically involves oral supplements of bicarbonate, potassium, and sodium.

3.   Type 3 RTA: This is a rare form of pediatric RTA and is caused by a defect in the kidney's ability to excrete acid. Children with type 3 RTA may experience symptoms such as growth retardation and rickets, a condition characterized by weak and brittle bones. Treatment for type 3 RTA typically involves oral supplements of bicarbonate and vitamin D to help promote bone growth and repair.

Diagnosis of RTA typically involves blood and urine tests to evaluate the body's acid-base balance and look for signs of kidney dysfunction. In some cases, a kidney biopsy may be necessary to determine the underlying cause of the RTA.

Treatment for RTA depends on the underlying cause and severity of the condition. In most cases, oral supplements of bicarbonate, potassium, and/or sodium can help restore the body's acid-base balance and prevent further complications. In severe cases, intravenous fluids or dialysis may be necessary.

Renal Tubular Acidosis can be a serious condition, with proper diagnosis and treatment, many children with RTA are able to manage their symptoms and prevent further complications. Regular monitoring and follow-up with a pediatric nephrologist is important for children with RTA to ensure the best possible outcomes.

Kidney Stones

Kidney stones are a relatively rare condition in children, but they can cause significant pain and discomfort when they do occur. Kidney stones are small, hard deposits of minerals and salts that form inside the kidneys and can block the flow of urine.

Symptoms of kidney stones in children may include:

- Severe pain in the back, side, or lower abdomen
- Painful or frequent urination
- Blood in the urine
- Nausea or vomiting
- Fever or chills (if an infection is present)

Causes of kidney stones in children can include dehydration, a diet high in salt or protein, certain medical conditions such as cystic fibrosis or hyperparathyroidism, and a family history of kidney stones.

Diagnosis of kidney stones typically involves a physical exam, urine and blood tests to look for signs of infection or kidney dysfunction, and imaging tests such as ultrasound or CT scan to visualize the stones in the kidneys and urinary tract.

Treatment for kidney stones may include:

1. Pain management: Severe pain caused by kidney stones can be managed with over-the-counter pain medications or prescription painkillers.
2. Fluids: Drinking plenty of fluids, particularly water, can help flush out the stones and prevent new ones from forming.
3. Medications: Certain medications, such as alpha-blockers or potassium citrate, may be prescribed to help relax the muscles in the urinary tract and prevent the formation of new stones.
4. Surgery: In some cases, surgical intervention may be

necessary to remove larger stones that cannot pass on their own.

Prevention of kidney stones in children includes encouraging a healthy diet and plenty of fluids to prevent dehydration. Children with a history of kidney stones may also benefit from regular monitoring and follow-up with a pediatric nephrologist to prevent recurrence.

Kidney stones can be a painful and uncomfortable condition, with proper diagnosis and treatment, most children are able to recover fully and prevent future occurrences.

CHAPTER 9

Infectious Disease

Pediatric infectious disease is a medical specialty that deals with the diagnosis and treatment of infectious diseases in children. Some of the common diagnoses that are treated by pediatric infectious disease specialists include:

1. Respiratory infections: These include infections of the upper respiratory tract, such as the common cold and flu, as well as lower respiratory tract infections such as pneumonia and bronchiolitis.

2. Gastrointestinal infections: These include infections of the digestive tract, such as gastroenteritis (stomach flu), rotavirus, and bacterial infections such as Salmonella, Shigella, and E. coli.

3. Skin infections: These include bacterial skin infections such as impetigo and cellulitis, viral infections such as chickenpox and warts, and fungal infections such as ringworm.

4. Urinary tract infections: These are infections of the urinary tract, including the bladder and kidneys, that can cause pain, fever, and other symptoms.

5. Bloodstream infections: These include sepsis, which is a serious infection that can spread throughout the body and cause organ failure.

6. Meningitis and encephalitis: These are infections of the

brain and spinal cord that can cause inflammation and other serious complications.

7.   Sexually transmitted infections: These include infections such as chlamydia, gonorrhea, and human papillomavirus (HPV).

8.   Lyme disease: This is a tick-borne illness that can cause fever, rash, and other symptoms.

9.   Tuberculosis: This is a bacterial infection that primarily affects the lungs, but can also affect other parts of the body.

10.   HIV/AIDS: This is a viral infection that attacks the immune system and can lead to serious complications if left untreated.

Treatment for these and other pediatric infectious disease diagnoses often includes a combination of medications, supportive care, and other specialized interventions, depending on the specific condition and individual needs of the child. Preventative measures such as vaccination and infection control practices are also important in the management of pediatric infectious diseases.

Respiratory Infections

Respiratory infections are a common occurrence in children, particularly during the fall and winter months. These infections can range from mild colds to more severe illnesses, such as pneumonia or bronchiolitis, and can be caused by a variety of viruses and bacteria.

Symptoms of respiratory infections in children can include:

- Runny or stuffy nose
- Cough
- Sore throat
- Fever
- Headache

- Fatigue
- Shortness of breath (in more severe cases)

Common types of respiratory infections include:

1. Common cold: The common cold is caused by a viral infection and can cause mild to moderate symptoms such as runny nose, cough, and sore throat. It typically resolves on its own within a week or two.
2. Influenza (flu): Influenza is a viral infection that can cause more severe symptoms such as high fever, body aches, and fatigue. It can be particularly dangerous in young children and may require antiviral medication and supportive care.
3. Bronchiolitis: Bronchiolitis is a viral infection that affects the small airways in the lungs and can cause wheezing, coughing, and difficulty breathing. It is most common in infants and young children.
4. Pneumonia: Pneumonia is a bacterial or viral infection of the lungs that can cause fever, cough, chest pain, and difficulty breathing. It can be particularly dangerous in young children and may require hospitalization and antibiotic treatment.
5. Croup: Croup is a viral infection that affects the upper airways and can cause a barking cough, hoarseness, and difficulty breathing. It is most common in young children and may require supportive care and sometimes steroid medication.

Treatment for respiratory infections may include:

1. Symptomatic treatment: Many respiratory infections are caused by viruses and do not respond to antibiotics. Symptomatic treatment may include over-the-counter pain and fever relievers, rest, and plenty of fluids.
2. Antiviral medication: In cases of influenza, antiviral medication may be prescribed to help reduce symptoms

BRIAN WALTER TEMPLE M.D.

and shorten the duration of illness.

3. Antibiotics: In cases of bacterial respiratory infections, such as pneumonia, antibiotics may be necessary to treat the infection.

4. Supportive care: Children with more severe respiratory infections may require hospitalization and supportive care such as oxygen therapy or mechanical ventilation.

Prevention of respiratory infections includes good hand hygiene, avoiding close contact with people who are sick, and ensuring children are up to date on their vaccinations. In addition, it is important to keep children away from secondhand smoke and to encourage healthy habits such as regular exercise and a balanced diet to support a strong immune system.

While respiratory infections can be a common and uncomfortable condition in children, most children recover fully with appropriate treatment and prevention strategies.

Gastrointestinal Infections

Pediatric gastrointestinal infections are common in children and are caused by a variety of bacteria, viruses, and parasites. These infections can range from mild diarrhea to more severe illnesses such as dysentery or gastroenteritis.

Symptoms of pediatric gastrointestinal infections can include:

- Diarrhea
- Vomiting
- Nausea
- Stomach pain or cramping
- Fever
- Dehydration

224

Common types of pediatric gastrointestinal infections include:

1. Rotavirus: Rotavirus is a highly contagious virus that can cause severe diarrhea and vomiting in young children. It is most common in infants and young children, and can be prevented by vaccination.
2. Norovirus: Norovirus is a highly contagious virus that can cause diarrhea, vomiting, and stomach pain. It is most common in children and can spread quickly in schools and daycare settings.
3. Salmonella: Salmonella is a type of bacteria that can cause food poisoning and gastrointestinal infections. It is commonly found in contaminated food and can cause diarrhea, fever, and stomach pain.
4. E. coli: E. coli is a type of bacteria that can cause gastrointestinal infections and food poisoning. It is commonly found in contaminated food or water and can cause diarrhea, stomach pain, and fever.
5. Giardia: Giardia is a parasite that can cause diarrhea and other gastrointestinal symptoms. It is commonly found in contaminated water sources such as streams, lakes, and swimming pools.

Treatment for pediatric gastrointestinal infections may include:

1. Fluid replacement: It is important to replace fluids lost through diarrhea and vomiting to prevent dehydration. This can be done by giving children oral rehydration solutions or intravenous fluids in severe cases.
2. Symptomatic treatment: Over-the-counter medications such as anti-diarrheals and antiemetics may be used to relieve symptoms of diarrhea and vomiting.

3.   Antibiotics: In cases of bacterial infections such as salmonella or E. coli, antibiotics may be necessary to treat the infection.

4.   Prevention strategies: Good hygiene practices such as frequent hand washing, proper food handling and storage, and avoiding contaminated water sources can help prevent pediatric gastrointestinal infections.

In some cases, gastrointestinal infections can lead to complications such as dehydration, malnutrition, or a weakened immune system. It is important to seek medical attention if symptoms persist or worsen, or if there are signs of dehydration such as decreased urine output or dry mouth.

While gastrointestinal infections can be uncomfortable and disruptive to daily life, most children recover fully with appropriate treatment and prevention strategies.

Skin Infections

Pediatric skin infections are a common problem in children and can range from mild conditions such as diaper rash to more serious infections such as cellulitis or impetigo. These infections can be caused by a variety of bacteria, viruses, and fungi and can affect any part of the skin.

Symptoms of pediatric skin infections can include:

- Redness
- Swelling
- Pain or tenderness
- Itching
- Rash or blisters
- Fever

Common types of pediatric skin infections include:

1.   Impetigo: Impetigo is a common bacterial skin infection

that can cause red, itchy sores that may ooze or crust over. It is most common in young children and can be treated with topical or oral antibiotics.

2. Cellulitis: Cellulitis is a bacterial infection that affects the deeper layers of the skin and can cause redness, swelling, and pain. It can be caused by several different types of bacteria and may require treatment with oral or intravenous antibiotics.

3. Ringworm: Ringworm is a fungal infection that can cause a ring-shaped rash on the skin. It is most common in children and can be treated with antifungal medication.

4. Scabies: Scabies is a contagious skin infestation caused by tiny mites that burrow into the skin. It can cause intense itching and a rash and is treated with prescription topical or oral medications.

5. Herpes simplex: Herpes simplex is a viral infection that can cause cold sores or genital herpes in children. It is typically treated with antiviral medication.

Treatment for pediatric skin infections may include:

1. Topical medication: Many mild skin infections can be treated with topical medications such as creams, ointments, or lotions.

2. Oral medication: More severe infections may require treatment with oral antibiotics or antifungal medications.

3. Home care: Some skin infections such as diaper rash can be treated with home remedies such as gentle cleansing and the use of diaper rash creams or ointments.

4. Prevention strategies: Good hygiene practices such as frequent hand washing and avoiding contact with infected individuals can help prevent the spread of skin infections.

In some cases, pediatric skin infections can lead to complications such as scarring or the spread of the infection to other parts of the body. It is important to seek medical attention if symptoms persist or worsen, or if there are signs of a more serious infection such as fever or spreading redness.

Pediatric skin infections can be uncomfortable and disruptive to daily life, most children recover fully with appropriate treatment and prevention strategies.

Bloodstream Infections

Bloodstream infections (BSIs) are a significant cause of morbidity and mortality in children, particularly in neonates and infants. BSIs are defined as the presence of bacteria, fungi, or other microorganisms in the bloodstream, which can cause severe systemic illness.

Causes: The most common cause of BSIs is bacterial infections, such as Staphylococcus aureus, Streptococcus pneumoniae, and Escherichia coli. However, fungal infections, such as Candida species, are also a significant cause of BSIs in immunocompromised children.
Risk factors:

Several factors can increase the risk of BSIs in children, including prematurity, immunocompromised status, the presence of a central venous catheter, prolonged hospitalization, and prior antibiotic exposure.

Symptoms: Symptoms of BSIs can vary depending on the age of the child, the underlying cause of the infection, and the severity of the illness. Infants and neonates may present with nonspecific symptoms, such as fever, lethargy, poor feeding, and respiratory distress. Older children may present with fever, chills, malaise, and signs of sepsis, such as tachycardia, hypotension, and altered mental status.

Diagnosis: The diagnosis of BSIs requires blood culture, which is the gold standard for identifying microorganisms in the bloodstream. Other diagnostic tests, such as chest X-rays, urine culture, and cerebrospinal fluid analysis, may also be necessary to identify the source of the infection.

Treatment: The treatment of BSIs involves the administration of appropriate antibiotics or antifungal agents. The choice of antimicrobial therapy depends on the suspected pathogen and the susceptibility profile of the microorganism. In addition, supportive care, such as fluid and electrolyte management, may be necessary to manage complications associated with BSIs.

Prevention: PreventingBSIs requires a multifaceted approach that includes the use of appropriate infection control measures, such as hand hygiene, environmental cleaning, and the appropriate use of antibiotics. Strategies to reduce the risk of central line-associated bloodstream infections, such as the use of chlorhexidine skin antiseptic and daily assessment of line necessity, are also essential in preventing BSIs.

Bloodstream infections are a significant cause of morbidity and mortality in children, particularly in neonates and infants. Early recognition, prompt diagnosis, and appropriate antimicrobial therapy are crucial in managing BSIs in children. Additionally, strategies to prevent BSIs, such as infection control measures and the appropriate use of antibiotics, are essential in reducing the incidence of BSIs in pediatric patients.

Meningitis and Encephalitis

Meningitis and encephalitis are two severe neurological conditions that can affect children. Meningitis is the inflammation of the protective membranes covering the brain and spinal cord, while encephalitis is the inflammation of the brain tissue itself.

Causes: The most common cause of meningitis and encephalitis in children is a viral infection. However, bacterial infections, such as Streptococcus pneumoniae and Neisseria meningitidis, can also cause meningitis. Other potential causes include fungal infections, parasitic infections, and autoimmune disorders.

Symptoms: The symptoms of meningitis and encephalitis can vary depending on the age of the child and the underlying cause of the infection. Infants may present with nonspecific symptoms, such as fever, irritability, poor feeding, and lethargy. Older children may present with more specific symptoms, such as headache, neck stiffness, photophobia, and altered mental status. In severe cases, seizures, coma, and even death can occur.

Diagnosis: The diagnosis of meningitis and encephalitis requires a thorough physical examination, as well as laboratory and imaging tests. Lumbar puncture, which involves taking a sample of cerebrospinal fluid (CSF), is the gold standard for diagnosing meningitis and encephalitis. Other tests, such as blood cultures, CT scan, and MRI, may also be necessary to identify the underlying cause of the infection.

Treatment: The treatment of meningitis and encephalitis involves the administration of appropriate antimicrobial or antiviral therapy. The choice of therapy depends on the suspected pathogen and the sensitivity profile of the microorganism. In addition, supportive care, such as fluid and electrolyte management, may be necessary to manage complications associated with these conditions.

Prevention: Preventing meningitis and encephalitis requires a multifaceted approach that includes vaccination against bacterial and viral pathogens, such as Haemophilus influenzae type b, Streptococcus pneumoniae, and measles. Additionally, the appropriate use of antibiotics and antiviral medications can help reduce the risk of these infections. In some cases, infection control measures, such as isolation and quarantine, may also be necessary to prevent the spread of infection.

Meningitis and encephalitis are two severe neurological conditions that can cause significant morbidity and mortality in children. Early recognition, prompt diagnosis, and appropriate antimicrobial or antiviral therapy are crucial in managing these conditions. Additionally, strategies to prevent these infections, such as vaccination and infection control measures, are essential in reducing the incidence of meningitis and encephalitis in pediatric patients.

Sexually Transmitted Diseases

Pediatric sexually transmitted diseases (STDs) are infections that are spread through sexual contact and can affect children and adolescents. While uncommon, the incidence of STDs in children is increasing, particularly in adolescents.

Types of STDs: There are several types of STDs that can affect children and adolescents, including:

1. Human papillomavirus (HPV): HPV is a common STD that can cause genital warts and increase the risk of cervical cancer in women.
2. Chlamydia: Chlamydia is a bacterial infection that can cause discharge and pain during urination.
3. Gonorrhea: Gonorrhea is a bacterial infection that can cause discharge and pain during urination.
4. Herpes simplex virus (HSV): HSV is a viral infection that can cause genital ulcers and cold sores.
5. Syphilis: Syphilis is a bacterial infection that can cause sores, rashes, and fever.

Risk factors: Children and adolescents who engage in sexual

activity, particularly unprotected sexual activity, are at increased risk of developing STDs. Other risk factors include a history of sexual abuse, multiple sexual partners, and a history of STDs.

Symptoms: The symptoms of STDs can vary depending on the type of infection and the age of the child. Some children may not have any symptoms at all, while others may have discharge, pain during urination, sores, or rashes in the genital area.

Diagnosis and treatment: The diagnosis of STDs requires a thorough physical examination, as well as laboratory testing. Treatment of pediatric STDs typically involves the administration of antibiotics or antiviral medications, depending on the type of infection. In addition, counseling and education on safe sexual practices and prevention of STDs may be necessary.

Prevention: Preventing STDs involves education and counseling on safe sexual practices and the prevention of sexually transmitted infections. This includes the use of condoms, abstinence, and regular STD testing. Additionally, parents and caregivers should be aware of the signs and symptoms of sexual abuse and report any concerns to healthcare providers or law enforcement.

Sexually transmitted diseases are infections that can affect children and adolescents who engage in sexual activity. Prevention and education on safe sexual practices and the prevention of STDs are essential in reducing the incidence of pediatric STDs. Early recognition, diagnosis, and treatment are crucial in managing these infections and preventing complications.

Lyme Disease

Lyme disease is a bacterial infection caused by the Borrelia burgdorferi bacterium, which is transmitted to humans through the bite of infected black-legged ticks (also known as deer ticks). Children are particularly susceptible to Lyme disease, and it can cause significant morbidity if left untreated.

Symptoms: The symptoms of Lyme disease can vary depending on the stage of the infection. Early symptoms may include fever, headache, fatigue, and a characteristic rash known as erythema migrans. Later symptoms may include joint pain, muscle pain, neurological symptoms, and heart palpitations.

Diagnosis: The diagnosis of Lyme disease requires a thorough physical examination, as well as laboratory testing. Blood tests, such as the enzyme-linked immunosorbent assay (ELISA) and Western blot, can be used to detect antibodies to the Borrelia burgdorferi bacterium. In some cases, imaging tests, such as magnetic resonance imaging (MRI) or computed tomography (CT) scans, may also be necessary to evaluate the extent of the infection.

Treatment: The treatment of Lyme disease typically involves the administration of antibiotics, such as doxycycline, amoxicillin, or cefuroxime. The duration and type of antibiotics depend on the stage of the infection and the age of the child. In some cases, hospitalization may be necessary to manage severe symptoms, such as neurological complications or heart problems.
Prevention:

Preventing Lyme disease involves avoiding tick bites and promptly removing ticks if they are found on the skin. This can be achieved by wearing protective clothing, such as long pants and sleeves, and using insect repellents that contain DEET or picaridin. Additionally, parents and caregivers should check children and pets for ticks after outdoor activities, especially in wooded or grassy areas.

In conclusion, Lyme disease is a bacterial infection that can cause significant morbidity in children if left untreated. Early recognition, diagnosis, and treatment are crucial in managing this infection and preventing complications. Prevention, including avoiding tick bites and prompt removal of ticks, is essential in reducing the incidence of pediatric Lyme disease.

Tuberculosis

Tuberculosis (TB) is a bacterial infection caused by Mycobacterium tuberculosis that primarily affects children under the age of 15. It is a significant public health problem, particularly in low- and middle-income countries. Children with TB can have a range of symptoms, and the disease can be difficult to diagnose and treat.

Symptoms: The symptoms of TB can vary depending on the age of the child and the severity of the infection. Common symptoms include coughing, fever, weight loss, poor appetite, night sweats, and fatigue. In some cases, children may also experience chest pain, shortness of breath, or difficulty breathing.

Diagnosis: The diagnosis of TB requires a thorough physical examination, as well as laboratory testing. The tuberculin skin test (also known as the Mantoux test) is commonly used to screen for TB in children. This involves injecting a small amount of purified protein derivative (PPD) under the skin and measuring the size of the resulting reaction after 48-72 hours. If the skin test is positive, additional testing may be necessary, such as a chest x-ray or sputum culture. In addition to skin testing, blood tests, such as quantiferon gold are becoming more available and less expensive.

Treatment: The treatment of TB typically involves a combination of antibiotics, such as isoniazid, rifampin, and pyrazinamide, for a period of 6-9 months. The exact duration and type of antibiotics depend on the severity of the infection and the child's age and weight. Treatment is typically provided under the supervision of a healthcare provider and may require hospitalization in severe cases.

Prevention: Preventing TB involves identifying and treating TB in adults who may be in close contact with children, such as parents, caregivers, or household members. This can be achieved through contact tracing and targeted screening programs. Additionally, vaccination with the Bacillus Calmette-Guérin (BCG) vaccine has been shown to be effective in reducing the incidence of TB in children, particularly in low- and middle-income countries.

Tuberculosis is a bacterial infection that primarily affects children under the age of 15. Early recognition, diagnosis, and treatment are crucial in managing this infection and preventing complications. Prevention, including identifying and treating TB in adults and vaccination with the BCG vaccine, is essential in reducing the incidence of pediatric TB.

HIV/AIDS

HIV/AIDS is a viral infection caused by the human immunodeficiency virus (HIV) that primarily affects children under the age of 15. HIV is transmitted through contact with infected bodily fluids, such as blood, semen, vaginal secretions, and breast milk. Children with HIV/AIDS can have a range of symptoms, and the disease can be difficult to diagnose and treat.

Symptoms: The symptoms of HIV/AIDS can vary depending on the age of the child and the severity of the infection. Infants and young children may have nonspecific symptoms, such as failure to thrive, recurrent infections, and developmental delays. Older children may experience symptoms such as fever, weight loss, fatigue, and swollen lymph nodes. In some cases, children may also experience neurological symptoms or opportunistic infections, such as pneumonia, tuberculosis, or candidiasis.

Diagnosis: The diagnosis of HIV/AIDS requires a thorough physical examination, as well as laboratory testing. HIV antibody testing is the most commonly used diagnostic test for HIV infection. In some cases, additional testing, such as viral load testing or CD4+ cell count, may be necessary to determine the severity of the infection.

Treatment: The treatment of HIV/AIDS typically involves a combination of antiretroviral therapy (ART) and supportive care. ART consists of a combination of drugs that work to suppress the virus and prevent it from replicating in the body. The exact type and duration of ART depend on the child's age, weight, and the severity of the infection. Supportive care may include treatment for opportunistic infections, as well as nutritional and psychosocial support.

Prevention: Preventing HIV/AIDS involves preventing mother-to-child transmission (MTCT) of HIV. This can be achieved through a range of interventions, including antiretroviral treatment for pregnant women, elective cesarean delivery, and avoidance of breastfeeding. Additionally, HIV testing and counseling programs can help to identify HIV-positive women and ensure that they receive appropriate care and treatment.

HIV/AIDS is a viral infection that primarily affects children under the age of 15. Early recognition, diagnosis, and treatment are crucial in managing this infection and preventing complications. Prevention, including interventions to prevent mother-to-child transmission and HIV testing and counseling programs, is essential in reducing the incidence of HIV/AIDS.

CHAPTER 10

Dermatology

Pediatric dermatology is a specialty that focuses on the diagnosis and treatment of skin, hair, and nail conditions in children. Common diagnoses treated by pediatric dermatologists include:

1. Eczema: Eczema is a chronic skin condition that causes itchy, red, and inflamed skin. It is a common condition in children and can be managed with topical creams, oral medications, and lifestyle modifications.
2. Acne: Acne is a common skin condition that affects many teenagers. It is characterized by pimples, blackheads, and whiteheads and can be treated with topical and oral medications.
3. Birthmarks: Birthmarks are areas of discolored skin that are present at birth or develop shortly after. They can be categorized into two main types: vascular birthmarks and pigmented birthmarks. Treatment options depend on the type and location of the birthmark.
4. Psoriasis: Psoriasis is a chronic skin condition that causes red, scaly patches on the skin. It can be treated with topical medications, phototherapy, and oral medications.
5. Warts: Warts are caused by a virus and can appear anywhere on the body. Treatment options include topical medications, freezing, and surgical removal.
6. Hair and scalp conditions: Pediatric dermatologists also

treat conditions that affect the hair and scalp, including alopecia areata (hair loss), dandruff, and scalp psoriasis.

7.   Skin infections: Skin infections, such as impetigo, folliculitis, and cellulitis, are common in children and can be treated with topical and oral antibiotics.

8. Skin allergies: Pediatric dermatologists also diagnose and treat skin allergies, including allergic contact dermatitis, atopic dermatitis, and urticaria (hives).

9.   Hemangiomas: Hemangiomas are benign tumors that are made up of blood vessels. They can appear on the skin or internal organs and can be treated with medication, laser therapy, or surgical removal.

Pediatric dermatologists provide comprehensive care for children with a wide range of skin, hair, and nail conditions, helping to improve the child's quality of life and prevent long-term complications.

Eczema

Eczema, also known as atopic dermatitis, is a common skin condition that affects children. It is a chronic and inflammatory disorder that causes dry, itchy, and scaly patches on the skin. The exact cause of eczema is unknown, but it is thought to be related to an overactive immune system response to certain triggers, such as allergens or irritants.

Symptoms: The symptoms of eczema can vary depending on the age of the child and the severity of the condition. Infants may develop a rash on their face, scalp, and neck, while older children may develop patches of dry, itchy, and scaly skin on their hands, feet, elbows, and knees. The affected areas may be red, inflamed, and ooze fluid in severe cases. The symptoms of eczema can be exacerbated by environmental factors, such as heat, humidity, and exposure to certain allergens or irritants.

Diagnosis: The diagnosis of eczema is typically based on a physical examination of the affected skin. The healthcare provider may also take a medical history to identify any potential triggers or underlying conditions that may be contributing to the child's symptoms. In some cases, additional testing, such as allergy testing, may be necessary to identify any specific allergens that may be triggering the child's symptoms.

Treatment: The treatment of eczema typically involves a combination of skin care and medication. Skin care measures may include avoiding irritants, keeping the skin moisturized, and using mild soaps and detergents. Topical corticosteroids, such as hydrocortisone, may be prescribed to reduce inflammation and relieve itching. In severe cases, oral corticosteroids or immunosuppressants may be necessary. Additionally, phototherapy, which involves exposing the skin to controlled amounts of UV light, may be beneficial in some cases.

Prevention: Preventing eczema involves identifying and avoiding potential triggers, such as allergens or irritants. This may include avoiding certain foods, using mild soaps and detergents, and keeping the skin moisturized. Additionally, regular bathing and moisturizing can help to reduce the risk of developing eczema.

Pediatric eczema is a chronic and inflammatory skin condition that causes dry, itchy, and scaly patches on the skin. Early recognition, diagnosis, and treatment are crucial in managing this condition and preventing complications. Prevention, including identifying and avoiding potential triggers, regular bathing and moisturizing, and using mild soaps and detergents, is essential in reducing the incidence of eczema.

Acne

Acne is a common skin condition that affects children and adolescents. It occurs when hair follicles become clogged with oil and dead skin cells, leading to the formation of pimples, blackheads, and whiteheads. Acne can occur on the face, neck, chest, back, and shoulders, and it can have a significant impact on a child's self-esteem.

Symptoms: The symptoms of acne can vary depending on the severity of the condition. Mild acne may manifest as whiteheads, blackheads, or small pimples, while more severe acne may lead to the formation of larger pimples, cysts, or nodules. Acne can also cause inflammation, redness, and scarring, particularly if it is not treated promptly.

Diagnosis: The diagnosis of acne is typically based on a physical examination of the affected skin. The healthcare provider may also take a medical history to identify any potential triggers or underlying conditions that may be contributing to the child's symptoms.

Treatment: The treatment of acne typically involves a combination of skin care and medication. Skin care measures may include washing the affected areas with a gentle cleanser, avoiding harsh soaps and scrubs, and using non-comedogenic moisturizers and sunscreens. Topical treatments, such as benzoyl peroxide, retinoids, and topical antibiotics, may be prescribed to reduce inflammation and prevent the formation of new pimples. In severe cases, oral antibiotics or isotretinoin may be necessary. Additionally, certain cosmetic procedures, such as chemical peels or light therapy, may be beneficial in some cases.
Prevention:

Preventing acne involves adopting healthy skin care habits, such as washing the face twice daily with a gentle cleanser, avoiding picking or squeezing pimples, and avoiding using oily or greasy cosmetics. Additionally, regular exercise and a healthy diet may help to reduce the risk of developing acne.

Acne is a common skin condition that affects children and adolescents. Early recognition, diagnosis, and treatment are crucial in managing this condition and preventing complications, such as scarring. Prevention, including adopting healthy skin care habits and maintaining a healthy lifestyle, is essential in reducing the incidence of pediatric acne.

Birthmarks

Birthmarks are common skin conditions that are present at birth or appear shortly after birth. They are usually harmless, but some types of birthmarks may require medical attention. There are two main types of pediatric birthmarks: vascular birthmarks and pigmented birthmarks.

1. Vascular birthmarks: Vascular birthmarks occur due to abnormalities in the blood vessels in the skin. They are usually red or pink in color, and their appearance can change over time. The most common types of vascular birthmarks are:

a. Strawberry hemangioma: This is a common type of birthmark that occurs in 5-10% of infants. It appears as a bright red, raised, and bumpy lesion that can grow rapidly in the first few months of life. It usually disappears by the age of 7.

b. Port-wine stain: This is a flat, pink or reddish-purple birthmark that appears on the face or neck. It can darken over time and may become more prominent with age. Port-wine stains are usually permanent.

c. Salmon patch or stork bite: These are flat, pink birthmarks that appear on the forehead, eyelids, or back of the neck. They are usually temporary and disappear within the first year of life.

2.   Pigmented birthmarks: Pigmented birthmarks occur due to an overgrowth of pigment cells in the skin. They can vary in color from light brown to black. The most common types of pigmented birthmarks are:

a. Mongolian spot: This is a blue-gray birthmark that appears on the lower back or buttocks of infants. It is common in babies with darker skin tones and usually fades by the age of 2.

b. Café-au-lait spot: This is a light brown birthmark that can appear anywhere on the body. It is usually oval in shape and can vary in size. Café-au-lait spots are often associated with neurofibromatosis, a genetic disorder that causes tumors to grow on nerves.

c. Congenital melanocytic nevus: This is a dark brown or black birthmark that can be present at birth or appear in the first few months of life. It can vary in size and may have a rough or bumpy texture. Larger congenital melanocytic nevi have a higher risk of developing into melanoma, a type of skin cancer.

Treatment of pediatric birthmarks depends on the type and severity of the birthmark. In some cases, no treatment is needed as the birthmark will fade or disappear on its own. However, if the birthmark is causing functional problems or affecting the child's self-esteem, treatment options may include laser therapy, surgical excision, or medication. It is important to consult a dermatologist or pediatrician if you have concerns about your child's birthmark.

Psoriasis

Psoriasis is a chronic autoimmune disorder that affects the skin, nails, and joints. It is characterized by the rapid growth of skin cells that results in thick, scaly, and itchy patches on the skin. The condition can occur at any age, but it is rare in infants and young children. Here are some details about pediatric psoriasis:

1.   Symptoms: The symptoms of psoriasis can vary depending on the type of psoriasis. The most common symptoms include:

a. Red, raised, and scaly patches on the skin
b. Itching, burning, or soreness in the affected areas
c. Dry and cracked skin that may bleed
d. Nail changes such as thickening, pitting, or separation from the nail bed

e. Joint pain, stiffness, and swelling in some cases

2. Causes: The exact cause of psoriasis is not known, but it is believed to be related to an immune system malfunction. In psoriasis, the immune system mistakenly attacks healthy skin cells, causing them to grow rapidly and accumulate on the surface of the skin. The condition can be triggered by several factors, including:

a. Genetics: Psoriasis tends to run in families, indicating a genetic predisposition to the condition.

b. Environmental factors: Certain environmental factors, such as stress, infections, injuries to the skin, and cold weather, can trigger psoriasis flare-ups.

c. Medications: Some medications, such as lithium, beta-blockers, and antimalarials, can trigger or worsen psoriasis symptoms.

3.   Diagnosis: Diagnosing psoriasis can be challenging

as the symptoms may resemble other skin conditions. A dermatologist will perform a physical exam and take a medical history to rule out other possible causes. They may also perform a skin biopsy to confirm the diagnosis.

4.   Treatment: There is no cure for psoriasis, but there are several treatment options that can help manage the symptoms. The treatment plan will depend on the severity of the condition and the age of the child. Some common treatment options include:

a. Topical treatments: These are creams, ointments, and lotions that are applied directly to the affected areas to reduce inflammation, itching, and scaling.

b. Phototherapy: This involves exposing the skin to controlled amounts of ultraviolet light to slow down the growth of skin cells and reduce inflammation.

c. Systemic medications: These are prescription medications that are taken orally or by injection to suppress the immune system and reduce inflammation.

d. Lifestyle changes: Making certain lifestyle changes, such as reducing stress, avoiding triggers, and maintaining a healthy weight, can also help manage psoriasis symptoms.

Psoriasis is a chronic autoimmune disorder that can be challenging to diagnose and manage. Early detection and treatment can help prevent complications and improve the child's quality of life. It is important to consult a dermatologist or pediatrician if you suspect your child has psoriasis or any other skin condition.

Warts

Warts, also known as verrucae, are non-cancerous growths on the skin caused by the human papillomavirus (HPV) infection.

They can occur on any part of the body, but most commonly appear on the hands and feet. Here are some details about pediatric warts:

1. Symptoms: Pediatric warts can vary in appearance, depending on their location and type. The most common symptoms include:

a. Small, rough, and raised bumps on the skin
b. Gray or brownish in color with black dots
c. Pain or tenderness when walking or using the affected area
d. Spreading to other areas of the body or to other people

2. Causes: Warts are caused by the human papillomavirus (HPV), a common virus that infects the top layer of skin. The virus can enter the body through tiny cuts or breaks in the skin and can be easily transmitted through direct contact with an infected person or an object contaminated with the virus.

3. Diagnosis: Warts are usually diagnosed by a dermatologist based on their appearance and location. In some cases, a skin biopsy may be required to confirm the diagnosis.

4. Treatment: There are several treatment options available for warts, but they can be difficult to treat and may require multiple treatments. Some common treatment options include:

a. Over-the-counter treatments: These include salicylic acid solutions, patches, or gels that are applied directly to the warts to dissolve them over time.

b. Cryotherapy: This involves freezing the warts with liquid nitrogen to destroy the infected tissue.

c. Laser therapy: This involves using a laser to remove the warts by targeting the infected tissue.

d. Surgery: In some cases, surgical removal of the warts may be necessary, especially for large or stubborn warts.

e. Immunotherapy: This involves boosting the immune system's ability to fight the virus using topical creams or injections.

5.   Prevention: Preventing the spread of HPV is the best way to prevent pediatric warts. This can be done by:

a. Avoiding direct contact with infected persons or objects
b. Covering cuts or breaks in the skin with bandages
c. Wearing flip-flops or sandals in public showers or pools

d. Avoiding sharing personal items, such as towels, razors, or shoes.

Warts are a common skin condition caused by the human papillomavirus (HPV) infection. They can be difficult to treat and may require multiple treatments. Preventing the spread of HPV is the best way to prevent pediatric warts. It is important to consult a dermatologist or pediatrician if you suspect your child has warts or any other skin condition.

Hair and Scalp Conditions

Hair and scalp conditions can range from mild dandruff to severe infections. Here are some of the most common pediatric hair and scalp conditions:

1.   Dandruff: Dandruff is a common condition that causes white or yellow flakes to appear on the scalp and in the hair. It is caused by a yeast-like fungus that lives on the scalp. Dandruff can be treated with over-the-counter medicated shampoos that contain ingredients like salicylic acid or ketoconazole.
2.   Head lice: Head lice are tiny, parasitic insects that live on the scalp and feed on blood. They can cause intense

itching and irritation. Head lice can be treated with over-the-counter or prescription medicated shampoos, lotions, or creams that contain insecticides.

3.   Ringworm: Ringworm is a fungal infection that can affect the scalp, causing hair loss and scaly patches on the skin. Ringworm can be treated with prescription antifungal medications, which may be given orally or applied topically.

4.   Folliculitis: Folliculitis is an infection of the hair follicles that can occur on the scalp or other parts of the body. It is caused by bacteria or fungi and can cause red, swollen, and painful bumps on the scalp. Folliculitis can be treated with prescription antibiotics or antifungal medications.

5.   Tinea capitis: Tinea capitis is a fungal infection that affects the scalp and hair shafts. It can cause hair loss, scaly patches on the skin, and swollen lymph nodes. Tinea capitis can be treated with prescription antifungal medications, which may be given orally or applied topically.

6.   Alopecia areata: Alopecia areata is an autoimmune condition that causes hair loss on the scalp or other parts of the body. It can cause patchy or complete hair loss, and there is no known cure. Treatment may include corticosteroid injections, topical medications, or immunosuppressants.

7.   Seborrheic dermatitis: Seborrheic dermatitis is a common condition that can affect the scalp and other areas of the body. It causes red, scaly, and itchy patches on the skin, and can also cause dandruff. Seborrheic dermatitis can be treated with medicated shampoos, topical corticosteroids, or antifungal medications.

Skin Infections

Skin infections are common in children, and they can range from mild to severe. Some of the most common pediatric skin infections include:

1. Impetigo: Impetigo is a highly contagious bacterial infection that causes red, oozing sores on the face, hands, and feet. It is caused by Staphylococcus aureus or Streptococcus pyogenes bacteria and can be treated with antibiotics.

2. Cellulitis: Cellulitis is a bacterial skin infection that causes red, swollen, and tender skin. It can be caused by a variety of bacteria and can be treated with antibiotics.

3. Erysipelas: Erysipelas is a bacterial skin infection that causes red, raised, and painful lesions on the skin. It is caused by Streptococcus pyogenes bacteria and can be treated with antibiotics.

4. Folliculitis: Folliculitis is an infection of the hair follicles that can cause red, swollen, and painful bumps on the skin. It can be caused by bacteria or fungi and can be treated with antibiotics or antifungal medications.

5. Herpes simplex virus: Herpes simplex virus (HSV) is a viral infection that can cause cold sores or fever blisters around the mouth or nose. It can also cause genital herpes, which can be transmitted through sexual contact. HSV can be treated with antiviral medications.

6. Varicella zoster virus: Varicella zoster virus (VZV) is a viral infection that causes chickenpox in children. It can cause itchy, blister-like lesions on the skin, fever, and other symptoms. VZV can be prevented with the varicella vaccine.

7. Human papillomavirus: Human papillomavirus (HPV) is a viral infection that can cause warts on the skin or genitals. It can be transmitted through direct contact with an infected person or an object contaminated with the virus. HPV can be prevented with the HPV vaccine.

8. Scabies: Scabies is a parasitic skin infection caused by tiny mites that burrow into the skin. It can cause intense itching and a rash of small, red bumps. Scabies can be

treated with prescription medications.

Many skin infections are highly contagious, so it is important to take steps to prevent their spread, such as washing hands regularly, avoiding close contact with infected individuals, and keeping skin clean and dry. Treatment for pediatric skin infections may include antibiotics, antifungal medications, or antiviral medications, depending on the cause of the infection.

Skin Allergies

Skin allergies are common in children and can be caused by a variety of factors. Some of the most common skin allergies in children include:

1. Eczema: Eczema, also known as atopic dermatitis, is a chronic skin condition that causes dry, itchy, and inflamed skin. It is often triggered by allergens such as dust, pet dander, or certain foods.
2. Contact dermatitis: Contact dermatitis is a skin rash caused by contact with an allergen or irritant, such as poison ivy, certain metals, or fragrances. The rash can be itchy, red, and may blister or ooze.
3. Hives: Hives, also known as urticaria, are red, itchy bumps on the skin that can appear suddenly and disappear just as quickly. They are often caused by an allergic reaction to food, medication, or insect bites.
4. Allergic dermatitis: Allergic dermatitis is a skin rash caused by an allergic reaction to something that comes in contact with the skin, such as cosmetics, soaps, or clothing.
5. Angioedema: Angioedema is a condition that causes swelling in the deeper layers of the skin, usually around the eyes and mouth. It can be caused by an allergic reaction to food, medication, or insect bites.
6. Seborrheic dermatitis: Seborrheic dermatitis is a common skin condition that causes red, scaly patches

on the scalp, face, and other areas of the body. It can be triggered by stress, certain medications, or changes in weather.

7.   Pruritus: Pruritus is a condition that causes intense itching of the skin. It can be caused by a variety of factors, including allergies, skin infections, or underlying medical conditions.

Identification of skin allergy is needed in order to properly treat it. Your pediatrician or allergist can perform allergy testing to determine what allergens your child is allergic to. Treatment for pediatric skin allergies may include antihistamines, topical or oral steroids, or avoiding the allergen altogether. It is also important to take steps to prevent allergic reactions, such as washing hands regularly, avoiding contact with known allergens, and using hypoallergenic products.

Hemangiomas

Hemangiomas are benign tumors that develop in infants and young children. They are composed of blood vessels that grow abnormally and can appear anywhere on the body. Hemangiomas can range in size from a small dot to a large, raised bump and can be flat or raised. They are more common in girls and premature infants.

There are two types of hemangiomas: superficial and deep. Superficial hemangiomas are located in the top layers of the skin, while deep hemangiomas are located in the deeper layers of the skin and can be more difficult to treat.

Most hemangiomas appear within the first few weeks of life and continue to grow for several months before beginning to shrink and disappear on their own. The growth phase can last up to a year or more, with the shrinking phase typically lasting several years. Hemangiomas may cause problems if they are located near the eyes, nose, or mouth and can interfere with vision or breathing.

Treatment for hemangiomas depends on their location, size, and severity. Most hemangiomas do not require treatment and will resolve on their own. However, if a hemangioma is causing problems, there are several treatment options available, including:

1. Corticosteroids: Corticosteroids can be given orally or injected into the hemangioma to help reduce inflammation and shrink the tumor.
2. Beta-blockers: Beta-blockers, such as propranolol, can be used to help shrink the hemangioma.
3. Laser therapy: Laser therapy can be used to remove the hemangioma, especially if it is located in a visible area or causes significant cosmetic concerns.
4. Surgery: Surgery may be required for hemangiomas that are causing significant functional problems, such as those located near the eyes or mouth.

Most hemangiomas will resolve on their own without causing any long-term problems. However, it is important to have your child's hemangioma evaluated by a pediatrician or dermatologist to ensure proper monitoring and treatment, if necessary.

CHAPTER 11

Developmental and Behavioral Pediatrics

Pediatric developmental and behavioral pediatrics is a medical specialty that focuses on the evaluation, diagnosis, and treatment of developmental and behavioral disorders in children. Some of the common diagnoses that are treated by developmental and behavioral pediatricians include:

1. Autism spectrum disorder (ASD): This is a developmental disorder that affects communication, social interaction, and behavior.
2. Attention deficit hyperactivity disorder (ADHD): This is a common behavioral disorder that affects attention, impulsivity, and hyperactivity.
3. Learning disabilities: These are disorders that affect the ability to learn and process information, such as dyslexia and dyscalculia.
4. Intellectual disability: This is a developmental disorder that affects cognitive abilities and intellectual functioning.
5. Speech and language disorders: These are disorders that affect communication, including speech delay and stuttering.
6. Anxiety and mood disorders: These are disorders that affect emotions, such as anxiety, depression, and bipolar

disorder.

7. Conduct disorder: This is a behavioral disorder that involves aggression, rule-breaking, and other disruptive behaviors.

8. Tourette syndrome: This is a neurological disorder that involves involuntary movements and vocalizations, called tics.

9. Developmental delays: These are delays in achieving developmental milestones, such as crawling, walking, and talking.

10. Feeding and eating disorders: These are disorders that affect the ability to eat and swallow, such as feeding aversion and selective eating disorder.

Treatment for these and other pediatric developmental and behavioral diagnoses often includes a combination of therapies, such as behavioral therapy, speech and language therapy, and occupational therapy, as well as medications when appropriate. Parent education and support are also important components of treatment, as well as collaboration with other healthcare providers, such as educators and mental health professionals.

Autism Spectrum Disorder

Autism Spectrum Disorder (ASD) is a developmental disorder that affects social communication and interaction, as well as behavior and sensory processing. The term "spectrum" is used because ASD can present itself in a wide range of symptoms, severity, and abilities. The symptoms of ASD typically appear in early childhood and persist throughout the individual's life.

ASD is diagnosed based on behavioral and developmental

evaluations, as there is no specific medical test or blood test for diagnosis. The Diagnostic and Statistical Manual of Mental Disorders (DSM-5) provides a set of criteria for diagnosing ASD, which includes difficulties in social communication and interaction, repetitive behaviors, and restricted interests.

The following are some common features of ASD:

The causes of autism spectrum disorders are complex and often involve a combination of genetic, environmental, and psychological factors. Some potential causes include:

1. Genetics: Social Communication and Interaction: Individuals with ASD have difficulties with social interaction and communication. They may have difficulty initiating and maintaining conversations, understanding nonverbal cues such as facial expressions and body language, and may have trouble understanding sarcasm and figurative language.
2. Repetitive Behaviors and Restricted Interests: Individuals with ASD may exhibit repetitive behaviors such as hand flapping, rocking back and forth, or echolalia (repeating words or phrases). They may also have restricted interests or preoccupations with specific objects or topics.
3. Sensory Processing: Individuals with ASD may be oversensitive or under sensitive to sensory stimuli such as sounds, lights, textures, or tastes.
4. Cognitive and Learning Differences: Individuals with ASD may have difficulty with executive functioning, which includes planning, organizing, and prioritizing tasks. They may also have difficulty with academic tasks, such as reading, writing, and math.

ASD is considered a lifelong condition, but with early intervention, individuals with ASD can learn strategies and skills to help them manage their symptoms and improve their quality of life. Treatment options for ASD include behavioral interventions, such as Applied Behavior Analysis (ABA), speech therapy, occupational therapy,

Individual with ASD are unique, and their symptoms can vary widely. Some individuals may require significant support throughout their lives, while others may be able to live independently with minimal support. It is important to provide individualized support and interventions based on the needs and strengths of each person with ASD.

Attention Deficit Hyperactivity Disorder

Attention Deficit Hyperactivity Disorder (ADHD) is a neurodevelopmental disorder that affects both children and adults. ADHD is characterized by symptoms of inattention, hyperactivity, and impulsivity that interfere with daily functioning and development. The symptoms of ADHD can vary in their severity and presentation from individual to individual, and may change over time.

The following are some common features of ADHD:

1. Inattention: Individuals with ADHD may have difficulty sustaining attention, getting organized, completing tasks, following instructions, and keeping track of details.
2. Hyperactivity: Individuals with ADHD may be overly active or restless, and have difficulty sitting still, remaining quiet, and waiting their turn.
3. Impulsivity: Individuals with ADHD may act without thinking, interrupt others, and have difficulty controlling their impulses.
4. Emotional Dysregulation: Individuals with ADHD may have difficulty regulating their emotions, resulting in mood swings, anger, and frustration.

ADHD is typically diagnosed by a healthcare provider, such

as a pediatrician or psychiatrist, based on a comprehensive evaluation that includes clinical history, rating scales, and behavioral observations. There is no single test to diagnose ADHD.

Treatment for ADHD typically involves a combination of behavioral interventions and medication. Behavioral interventions may include parent training, behavioral therapy, and school-based interventions to improve academic and social functioning. Medications commonly used to treat ADHD include stimulant medications such as methylphenidate and amphetamines, and non-stimulant medications such as atomoxetine and guanfacine.

While medication can be an effective treatment for ADHD, it is not a cure. Behavioral interventions such as parent training and therapy are also important components of treatment, and can help individuals with ADHD learn strategies for managing their symptoms and improving their quality of life.

In addition to medication and behavioral interventions, individuals with ADHD may benefit from accommodations and support in school and work settings. These accommodations may include extended time on tests, preferential seating, and frequent breaks.

With proper treatment and support, individuals with ADHD can lead successful and fulfilling lives. However, it is important to seek professional help if you suspect you or a loved one may have ADHD, as early intervention can lead to better outcomes.

Learning Disabilities

Pediatric learning disabilities refer to a group of conditions that affect a child's ability to learn and process information. Learning disabilities are not related to intelligence or motivation, but rather result from differences in brain structure or function. The following are some common types of pediatric learning disabilities:

1. Dyslexia: Dyslexia is a learning disability that affects reading and language processing. Individuals with dyslexia may have difficulty recognizing words, reading fluently, and comprehending what they read.
2. Dyscalculia: Dyscalculia is a learning disability that affects mathematical processing. Individuals with dyscalculia may have difficulty with basic arithmetic, understanding mathematical concepts, and memorizing math facts.
3. Dysgraphia: Dysgraphia is a learning disability that affects writing and fine motor skills. Individuals with dysgraphia may have difficulty with handwriting, spelling, and organizing their thoughts on paper.
4. Nonverbal Learning Disability (NVLD): NVLD is a learning disability that affects social skills and spatial processing. Individuals with NVLD may have difficulty with nonverbal communication, interpreting facial expressions, and understanding spatial relationships.
5. Attention Deficit Hyperactivity Disorder (ADHD): ADHD is a neurodevelopmental disorder that affects attention, hyperactivity, and impulsivity. Children with ADHD may have difficulty with organization, following directions, and completing tasks.

Pediatric learning disabilities are typically diagnosed by a neuropsychologist or other healthcare provider who specializes in learning disabilities. The diagnosis process may involve a comprehensive evaluation that includes clinical history, cognitive and academic testing, and behavioral observations.

Treatment for pediatric learning disabilities typically involves a combination of academic support, behavioral interventions, and accommodations. Academic support may include specialized tutoring, educational therapy, and individualized educational plans (IEPs). Behavioral interventions may include parent training, cognitive-behavioral therapy, and social skills training. Accommodations may include extra time on tests, preferential seating, and assistive technology.

While children with learning disabilities may face challenges, they can still achieve academic and personal success with proper treatment and support. It is important to seek professional help if you suspect your child may have a learning disability, as early intervention can lead to better outcomes.

Intellectual Disability (ID)

Pediatric Intellectual Disability (ID), also known as intellectual developmental disorder, refers to a condition in which a child's cognitive and adaptive functioning is significantly below average. Children with ID may have difficulty with learning, problem-solving, and adaptive skills such as communication, self-care, and socialization.

The severity of ID can range from mild to severe, and is typically diagnosed based on the child's IQ score, which is measured by standardized tests of cognitive ability. The American Psychiatric Association's Diagnostic and Statistical Manual of Mental Disorders, Fifth Edition (DSM-5) defines ID as an IQ score of below 70, accompanied by limitations in adaptive functioning.

ID can result from a variety of causes, including genetic and chromosomal abnormalities, brain damage or injury, and environmental factors such as malnutrition or exposure to toxins. Some of the most common causes of ID include Down syndrome, Fragile X syndrome, and fetal alcohol syndrome.

Children with ID may also have co-occurring conditions, such as epilepsy, cerebral palsy, or autism spectrum disorder. These co-occurring conditions can further impact the child's development and quality of life.

Treatment for pediatric ID typically involves a multidisciplinary approach that addresses the child's individual needs and strengths. This may include special education services, individualized therapy, and behavioral interventions. For children with severe ID, residential treatment may be necessary.

Families and caregivers of children with ID should provide a supportive and nurturing environment that promotes the child's social, emotional, and cognitive development. This may involve specialized education programs, structured daily routines, and opportunities for social interaction and community engagement.

While ID can present significant challenges for children and their families, early intervention and appropriate treatment can help children with ID reach their full potential and lead fulfilling lives. It is important to seek professional help if you suspect your child may have ID, as early intervention can lead to better outcomes.

Speech and Language Disorders

Pediatric speech and language disorders refer to a range of conditions that affect a child's ability to communicate effectively. These disorders can have a significant impact on a child's social, emotional, and cognitive development, as well as their academic performance. In this response, we will discuss pediatric speech and language disorders in detail, including their symptoms, causes, and treatment options.

Symptoms of Pediatric Speech and Language Disorders:

The symptoms of speech and language disorders can vary depending on the type and severity of the disorder. Some common symptoms of these disorders include:

1. Delayed speech development: Children with speech and language disorders may have delayed speech development and difficulty expressing themselves verbally.
2. Limited vocabulary: Children with speech and language disorders may have a limited vocabulary and struggle to find the right words to express their thoughts and ideas.
3. Articulation difficulties: Children with speech and language disorders may have difficulty producing certain sounds or pronouncing words correctly, which can make it difficult for others to understand them.
4. Stuttering: Children with speech and language disorders may also experience stuttering or difficulty with the flow of speech.

Causes of Pediatric Speech and Language Disorders:The causes of speech and language disorders can be complex and multifactorial. Some common causes of these disorders include:

1. Neurological Conditions:Speech and language disorders can be caused by neurological conditions such as cerebral palsy, Down syndrome, or autism spectrum disorder.
2. Hearing Loss:Hearing loss can also contribute to speech and language disorders, as children may have difficulty hearing and processing speech sounds.
3. Environmental Factors:Environmental factors such as a lack of exposure to language, inadequate language stimulation, or neglect can also contribute to speech and language disorders.

Treatment of Pediatric Speech and Language Disorders:The treatment of speech and language disorders depends on the specific disorder and the underlying cause. Treatment options may include:

1. Speech Therapy:Speech therapy is the most common treatment for speech and language disorders. A speech therapist will work with the child to improve their communication skills through exercises and techniques designed to improve speech and language development.
2. Assistive Technology:Assistive technology, such as communication devices or hearing aids, may also be helpful in managing speech and language disorders.
3. Behavioral Therapy:Behavioral therapy, such as social skills training or cognitive-behavioral therapy, may be effective in addressing the emotional and social effects of speech and language disorders.
4. Educational Support:

Educational support, such as individualized education plans (IEPs) or accommodations in the classroom, can also help children with speech and language disorders succeed academically.

Pediatric speech and language disorders refer to a range of conditions that affect a child's ability to communicate effectively. The symptoms and causes of these disorders can vary, and the treatment options depend on the specific disorder and the underlying cause. Early intervention is essential to ensure the best outcomes for children with speech and language disorders, and it is important to seek professional help if you suspect that your child may be experiencing a speech or language disorder.

Anxiety and Mood Disorders

Pediatric anxiety and mood disorders are common mental health conditions that affect children and adolescents. These disorders can have a significant impact on a child's emotional, social, and academic functioning. In this response, we will discuss pediatric anxiety and mood disorders in detail, including their symptoms, causes, and treatment options.

Anxiety Disorders: Anxiety disorders are the most common mental health conditions in children and adolescents, affecting approximately 10-20% of youth. These disorders are characterized by excessive and persistent fear, worry, and anxiety that interfere with a child's daily activities. The most common types of anxiety disorders in children and adolescents include:

1. Generalized Anxiety Disorder (GAD): Children with GAD experience excessive and persistent worry about a variety of everyday events and activities. They may worry excessively about things like grades, health, safety, and the future. Children with GAD may also have physical symptoms such as headaches, stomach aches, and muscle tension.

2. Separation Anxiety Disorder: Separation anxiety disorder is characterized by excessive and persistent fear or anxiety about being separated from their parents or caregivers. Children with separation anxiety disorder may refuse to attend school, avoid sleepovers, and experience nightmares or other sleep disturbances.

3. Specific Phobias: Specific phobias involve an excessive and persistent fear of a particular object or situation. Common phobias in children include fear of animals, heights, and needles.

4. Social Anxiety Disorder: Social anxiety disorder is characterized by a persistent and intense fear of social situations. Children with social anxiety disorder may experience extreme shyness, avoidance of social situations, and physical symptoms such as blushing, sweating, and trembling.

Causes of Pediatric Anxiety Disorders:

1.Genetics: Research suggests that anxiety disorders can run in families. Children with a family history of anxiety disorders may be more likely to develop these conditions themselves.

2. Brain Chemistry: Some research suggests that imbalances in brain chemicals such as serotonin and dopamine may play a role in the development of anxiety disorders.

3. Trauma:Exposure to traumatic events such as abuse, neglect, or a natural disaster can increase a child's risk of developing an anxiety disorder.

4. Parenting Style:Children with overprotective or controlling parents may be more likely to develop anxiety disorders.

Treatment of Anxiety Disorders:The treatment of anxiety disorders typically involves a combination of therapy and medication. The most effective therapies for children with anxiety disorders are cognitive-behavioral therapy (CBT) and exposure therapy. Medications such as selective serotonin reuptake inhibitors (SSRIs) may also be prescribed to help manage symptoms.

Pediatric Mood Disorders: Mood disorders are a group of mental health conditions characterized by persistent and extreme changes in mood or emotion. These disorders can cause significant impairment in a child's daily functioning. The most common types of mood disorders in children and adolescents include:

1. Major Depressive Disorder: Major depressive disorder

is a condition characterized by persistent feelings of sadness, hopelessness, and loss of interest or pleasure in activities. Children with major depressive disorder may also experience physical symptoms such as fatigue, changes in appetite, and sleep disturbances.

2.   Bipolar Disorder: Bipolar disorder is a condition characterized by extreme shifts in mood, energy, and activity levels. Children with bipolar disorder may experience manic episodes, which involve feelings of extreme happiness, impulsivity, and high energy, followed by depressive episodes.

3.   Disruptive Mood Dysregulation Disorder: Disruptive mood dysregulation disorder is a condition characterized by frequent and severe temper tantrums that are out of proportion to the situation. Children with disruptive mood dysregulation disorder may also have a persistent irritable or angry mood most of the day, nearly every day.

Causes of Mood Disorders: Like anxiety disorders, the causes of pediatric mood disorders are complex and involve a combination of genetic, environmental, and psychological factors. Some potential causes include:

1.   Genetics: Research suggests that mood disorders can run in families. Children with a family history of mood disorders may be more likely to develop these conditions themselves.

2.   Brain Chemistry: Imbalances in brain chemicals such as serotonin, dopamine, and norepinephrine may play a role in the development of mood disorders.

3.   Environmental Factors: Stressful life events such as trauma, abuse, or neglect can increase a child's risk of developing a mood disorder.

4.   Parenting Style: Parenting style, including neglectful or inconsistent parenting, can increase a child's risk of developing a mood disorder.

Treatment of Pediatric Mood Disorders:

The treatment of mood disorders typically involves a combination of therapy and medication. The most effective therapies for children with mood disorders are cognitive-behavioral therapy (CBT) and family therapy. Medications such as antidepressants, mood stabilizers, and antipsychotics may also be prescribed to help manage symptoms.

Anxiety and mood disorders are common mental health conditions that can significantly impact a child's emotional, social, and academic functioning. It's essential to seek professional help if you suspect that your child may be struggling with an anxiety or mood disorder. Early diagnosis and treatment can improve outcomes and help your child lead a healthy, fulfilling life.

Conduct Disorders

Pediatric conduct disorder is a type of disruptive behavior disorder that affects children and adolescents. Children with conduct disorder typically exhibit persistent and repetitive patterns of behavior that violate the rights of others and societal norms. In this response, we will discuss pediatric conduct disorders in detail, including their symptoms, causes, and treatment options.

Symptoms of Conduct Disorder: The symptoms of pediatric conduct disorder can vary depending on the child's age and the severity of the condition. The primary symptoms of conduct disorder include:

1. Aggressive Behavior: Children with conduct disorder may exhibit aggressive behavior, such as physical fights, bullying, or intimidating others.
2. Violation of Rules: Children with conduct disorder often violate rules and laws, such as stealing, lying, and

skipping school.

3.   Impulsivity: Children with conduct disorder may act impulsively without considering the consequences of their actions.

4.   Lack of Empathy: Children with conduct disorder may have difficulty understanding and empathizing with others.

5.   Animal Cruelty: Some children with conduct disorder may exhibit cruelty to animals.

Causes of Conduct Disorder: The causes of pediatric conduct disorder are complex and involve a combination of genetic, environmental, and psychological factors. Some potential causes include:

1.   Genetics: Research suggests that conduct disorder can run in families, and there may be a genetic component to the condition.

2.   Environmental Factors: Exposure to poverty, neglect, abuse, and trauma can increase a child's risk of developing conduct disorder.

3.   Parenting Style: Children who grow up in homes with inconsistent or neglectful parenting may be more likely to develop conduct disorder.

4.   Brain Chemistry: Imbalances in brain chemicals such as serotonin and dopamine may contribute to the development of conduct disorder.

Treatment of Conduct Disorder: The treatment of pediatric conduct disorder typically involves a combination of therapy and medication. The most effective therapies for children with conduct disorder are cognitive-behavioral therapy (CBT) and family therapy. Medications such as antidepressants and antipsychotics may also be prescribed to help manage symptoms.

Tourette's Syndrome

Tourette's syndrome (TS) is a neurodevelopmental disorder characterized by repetitive, involuntary movements and vocalizations called tics. The disorder usually starts in childhood and affects more boys than girls. In this response, we will discuss pediatric Tourette's syndrome in detail, including its symptoms, causes, and treatment options.

Symptoms of Tourette's Syndrome: The primary symptoms of Tourette's syndrome are tics. These tics can be divided into two categories: motor tics and vocal tics.

1. Motor Tics: Motor tics are sudden, repetitive movements that are involuntary and difficult to control. Examples of motor tics include eye blinking, facial grimacing, head jerking, shoulder shrugging, and other complex movements.
2. Vocal Tics: Vocal tics are sudden, involuntary sounds or words that are difficult to control. Examples of vocal tics include throat clearing, grunting, sniffing, and saying words out of context.

Causes of Tourette's Syndrome: The exact causes of Tourette's syndrome are not known, but it is believed to be a combination of genetic, environmental, and neurological factors.

1. Genetics: Tourette's syndrome tends to run in families, and there may be a genetic component to the disorder.
2. Neurological Factors: Tourette's syndrome is believed to be caused by a problem with the basal ganglia, a part of the brain that controls movement.
3. Environmental Factors: Environmental factors, such as infections, trauma, and stress, may trigger the onset of Tourette's syndrome.

Treatment of Tourette's Syndrome: While there is no cure

for Tourette's syndrome, the symptoms can be managed with treatment. The most effective treatments for Tourette's syndrome are behavioral therapy, medication, and sometimes a combination of both.

1. Behavioral Therapy: Behavioral therapy can help children with Tourette's syndrome manage their tics and reduce the impact of the disorder on their daily life. Techniques such as habit reversal training and cognitive-behavioral therapy can be effective in managing tics.

2. Medication: Medications such as antipsychotics, antidepressants, and alpha-agonists can help manage the symptoms of Tourette's syndrome. These medications work by altering brain chemicals and reducing the frequency and intensity of tics.

Developmental Delays

Pediatric developmental delays refer to a significant delay or difference in a child's development compared to other children their age. These delays can affect a child's physical, cognitive, social, or emotional development. In this response, we will discuss pediatric developmental delays in detail, including their symptoms, causes, and treatment options.

Symptoms of Developmental Delays: The symptoms of developmental delays can vary depending on the area of development that is affected. Some common symptoms of developmental delays include:

1. Physical Development: Delays in physical development can include delayed gross motor skills such as crawling, walking, or running, as well as fine motor skills such as holding a pencil or cutting with scissors.

2. Cognitive Development: Delays in cognitive development

can include difficulties with language, memory, problem-solving, and learning.

3. Social and Emotional Development: Delays in social and emotional development can include difficulty with social interactions, making friends, and regulating emotions.

Causes of Developmental Delays: The causes of developmental delays can vary and can be due to genetic, environmental, or medical factors.

1. Genetic Factors: Some developmental delays can be caused by genetic factors, such as Down syndrome, Fragile X syndrome, or other genetic disorders.
2. Environmental Factors: Environmental factors such as malnutrition, neglect, exposure to toxins, or trauma can also contribute to developmental delays.
3. Medical Factors: Medical factors such as prematurity, low birth weight, or infections during pregnancy can also cause developmental delays.

Treatment of Developmental Delays: The treatment of developmental delays depends on the underlying cause and the specific area of development that is affected. Treatment options may include:

1. Therapy: Therapy can be an effective treatment for developmental delays. Occupational therapy, physical therapy, and speech therapy can help children develop the skills they need to function at their age-appropriate level.
2. Medication: In some cases, medication may be prescribed to manage symptoms related to developmental delays, such as attention deficit hyperactivity disorder (ADHD) or anxiety.
3. Early Intervention: Early intervention is essential for children with developmental delays. The earlier a child receives treatment, the more likely they are to make progress and catch up to their peers.

Pediatric developmental delays refer to a significant delay or difference in a child's development compared to other children their age. The symptoms and causes of developmental delays can vary, and the treatment options depend on the specific area of development that is affected. If you suspect that your child may be experiencing developmental delays, it is essential to seek professional help for an accurate diagnosis and appropriate treatment. Early intervention can improve outcomes and help your child reach their full potential.

Feeding and Eating Disorders

Pediatric feeding and eating disorders refer to a range of conditions that affect a child's ability to eat, digest, or absorb food properly. These disorders can have significant physical and psychological effects on a child's health and development. In this response, we will discuss pediatric feeding and eating disorders in detail, including their symptoms, causes, and treatment options.

Symptoms of Pediatric Feeding and Eating Disorders: The symptoms of feeding and eating disorders can vary depending on the type of disorder. Some common symptoms of these disorders include:

1. Refusal to eat: Children with feeding and eating disorders may refuse to eat or drink certain foods, textures, or tastes.
2. Sensory issues: Children with feeding and eating disorders may have sensory issues, such as difficulty tolerating certain textures, smells, or tastes.
3. Choking or gagging: Children with feeding and eating disorders may experience choking or gagging when eating or drinking.
4. Delayed development: Feeding and eating disorders can cause delayed growth and development due to inadequate

nutrition.

Causes of Feeding and Eating Disorders: The causes of feeding and eating disorders can be complex and multifactorial. Some common causes of these disorders include:

1. Medical Conditions: Feeding and eating disorders can be caused by medical conditions such as gastrointestinal issues, allergies, or sensory processing disorders.
2. Psychological Factors: Psychological factors such as anxiety, trauma, or a history of abuse can also contribute to feeding and eating disorders.
3. Environmental Factors: Environmental factors such as a lack of parental support, pressure to eat or body image issues can also contribute to feeding and eating disorders.

Treatment of Feeding and Eating Disorders: The treatment of feeding and eating disorders depends on the type of disorder and the underlying cause. Treatment options may include:

1. Behavioral Therapy: Behavioral therapy, such as cognitive-behavioral therapy or family-based therapy, can be effective in treating feeding and eating disorders.
2. Dietary Changes: Dietary changes, such as modifying the texture or consistency of foods, can help children with feeding and eating disorders overcome sensory issues and increase their tolerance for different foods.
3. Medication: In some cases, medication may be prescribed to manage symptoms related to feeding and eating disorders, such as anxiety or depression.
4. Nutritional Support: Nutritional support, such as tube feeding or intravenous (IV) nutrition, may be necessary for children with severe feeding and eating disorders to ensure adequate nutrition and promote healthy growth and development.

Feeding and eating disorders refer to a range of conditions that affect a child's ability to eat, digest, or absorb food properly.

The symptoms and causes of these disorders can vary, and the treatment options depend on the specific disorder and the underlying cause. If you suspect that your child may be experiencing a feeding or eating disorder, it is essential to seek professional help for an accurate diagnosis and appropriate treatment. Early intervention can improve outcomes and help your child achieve and maintain a healthy relationship with food.

CHAPTER 12

Urology

P ediatric urology is a surgical subspecialty that focuses on the diagnosis and treatment of urological conditions in children. Some of the common diagnoses treated by pediatric urologists include:

1. Hydronephrosis: This is a condition where there is swelling or enlargement of the kidney due to urine backup. It can be caused by an obstruction in the urinary tract, and treatment options include surgery or medication.

2. Undescended testes: This is a condition where one or both testicles do not descend into the scrotum. It is common in newborns and young children and can be treated with hormone therapy or surgery.

3. Urinary tract infections (UTIs): UTIs are common in children and can be caused by bacteria in the urinary tract. Treatment usually involves antibiotics.

4. Vesicoureteral reflux (VUR): VUR is a condition where urine flows backward from the bladder into the ureters and kidneys, which can lead to urinary tract infections and kidney damage. Treatment options include medication, surgery, or watchful waiting.

5. Bedwetting: Bedwetting is common in children and can be caused by a variety of factors. Treatment options include behavioral therapy, medication, and alarm

therapy.

6.   Ureteropelvic junction obstruction: This is a condition where there is a blockage at the junction of the ureter and the kidney, which can lead to hydronephrosis. Treatment options include surgery or observation.

7.   Bladder exstrophy: This is a rare congenital condition where the bladder is exposed on the outside of the body. Treatment usually involves surgery.

8.   Congenital anomalies of the kidney and urinary tract: These are a group of congenital conditions that affect the kidneys and urinary tract. Treatment options depend on the specific condition.

9.   Phimosis: This is a condition where the foreskin of the penis cannot be retracted. Treatment options include topical steroids or circumcision.

10. Hypospadias: Hypospadias is a congenital condition in which the urethral opening is located on the underside of the penis instead of at the tip.

11. Inguinal Hernia: Inguinal hernias occurs when a portion of intestine or other abdominal contents protrudes through a weakened area or opening in the abdominal wall near the groin

12. Penile Adhesions and Skin Bridges: Penile adhesions and skin bridges are conditions that involve the fusion or connection of the skin on the penis

13. Labile Adhesions: Also known as labial agglutination, occur when the inner labia of the female genitalia become stuck together.

Pediatric urologists provide comprehensive care for children with a wide range of urological conditions, helping to improve their quality of life and prevent long-term complications.

Hydronephrosis

Hydronephrosis is a condition that occurs when urine flow

from the kidney to the bladder is obstructed, leading to the accumulation of urine in the kidney. This can cause dilation or swelling of the kidney and ureter, and if left untreated, it can result in permanent damage to the kidney. In this response, we will discuss pediatric hydronephrosis in detail, including its causes, symptoms, diagnosis, and treatment options.

Causes: Hydronephrosis can be caused by a variety of factors, including:

1. Congenital abnormalities: These are defects that occur during fetal development, such as ureteropelvic junction (UPJ) obstruction, vesicoureteral reflux (VUR), or posterior urethral valves (PUV).
2. Neurogenic bladder: A neurogenic bladder is a condition in which there is a disruption of the normal nerve function that controls the bladder, leading to an inability to empty the bladder properly.
3. Tumors: Kidney or bladder tumors can cause obstruction and subsequent hydronephrosis.
4. Kidney stones: Stones that form in the kidney or ureter can cause obstruction and hydronephrosis.

Symptoms: The symptoms of pediatric hydronephrosis depend on the severity of the condition. Mild hydronephrosis may not cause any symptoms, while severe hydronephrosis can cause significant discomfort and pain. Some common symptoms include:

1. Abdominal or flank pain
2. Nausea and vomiting
3. Urinary tract infection
4. Hematuria (blood in the urine)
5. Poor growth or failure to thrive

Diagnosis: Hydronephrosis is usually diagnosed through imaging studies such as ultrasound, magnetic resonance imaging (MRI), or computed tomography (CT) scan. In some cases, a voiding cystourethrogram (VCUG) may be ordered to evaluate for vesicoureteral reflux (VUR). Blood tests may also be ordered to evaluate kidney function.

Treatment: The treatment of hydronephrosis depends on the underlying cause and severity of the condition. Mild hydronephrosis may not require treatment, while severe cases may require surgical intervention. Some common treatment options include:

1. Observation: Mild cases of hydronephrosis may be closely monitored with regular imaging studies to ensure that the condition does not worsen.
2. Antibiotics: If a urinary tract infection is present, antibiotics may be prescribed to treat the infection and prevent further damage to the kidney.
3. Surgery: In cases where there is a significant obstruction or blockage, surgery may be necessary to remove the obstruction and restore normal urine flow.
4. Drainage: In some cases, a percutaneous nephrostomy tube may be placed to drain the urine from the kidney and relieve pressure.

Hydronephrosis is a condition that requires prompt diagnosis and treatment to prevent permanent kidney damage. If your child experiences symptoms of hydronephrosis, it is important to seek medical attention as soon as possible.

Undescended Testes

Undescended testes, also known as cryptorchidism, is a common condition that occurs in male infants and young children. It refers to the failure of one or both testicles to descend into the scrotum during fetal development or within the first few months of life. In this response, we will discuss undescended testes in the pediatric population, including its causes, symptoms, diagnosis, and treatment options.

Causes: The exact cause of undescended testes is not known, but it is believed to be due to a combination of genetic and environmental factors. Some of the factors that may contribute to the condition include:

1. Hormonal imbalances: Hormones produced during fetal development are essential for the proper development and descent of the testicles. Any disruption in hormone production can lead to undescended testes.
2. Abnormalities in the development of the reproductive system: Certain abnormalities in the development of the reproductive system can prevent the testicles from descending into the scrotum.
3. Prematurity: Premature infants are more likely to have undescended testes than full-term infants.

Symptoms: Undescended testes may not cause any symptoms, but in some cases, it can cause discomfort, pain, or swelling in the groin area. It can also increase the risk of infertility and testicular cancer later in life.

Diagnosis: Undescended testes are usually diagnosed during a physical examination by a healthcare provider. The provider will look for the presence of the testicles in the scrotum and may perform an ultrasound to locate the testicles if they are not visible. Blood tests may also be ordered to evaluate hormone levels.

Treatment: The treatment of undescended testes depends on the age of the child and the severity of the condition. In most cases, treatment is recommended to prevent complications later in life. Some common treatment options include:

1. Observation: In some cases, undescended testes may descend on their own during the first few months of life. Regular follow-up appointments with a healthcare provider may be recommended to monitor the condition.
2. Hormone therapy: Hormone therapy may be used to

stimulate the descent of the testicles. This treatment is usually reserved for infants younger than 6 months of age.

3.   Surgery: If the testicles do not descend on their own or with hormone therapy, surgery may be necessary to move them into the scrotum. The surgery is usually performed between the ages of 6 and 12 months.

Undescended testes is a common condition that requires prompt diagnosis and treatment to prevent complications later in life.

Urinary Tract Infections (UTIs)

Urinary tract infections (UTIs) are a common infection in children, especially in infants and toddlers. It occurs when bacteria or other pathogens invade the urinary tract, which includes the kidneys, ureters, bladder, and urethra. In this response, we will discuss UTIs in the pediatric population, including its causes, symptoms, diagnosis, and treatment options.

Causes: UTIs in children are usually caused by bacteria that enter the urinary tract through the urethra. In some cases, the infection can occur when bacteria from the stool enter the urethra, such as when wiping after a bowel movement or from poor hygiene practices. Certain conditions, such as vesicoureteral reflux, can also increase the risk of UTIs in children.

Symptoms: The symptoms of UTIs in children can vary depending on the age of the child. Infants and young children may exhibit nonspecific symptoms such as:

1.   Fever
2.   Vomiting
3.   Irritability

4. Poor feeding
5. Failure to thrive

Older children may experience symptoms similar to adults, such as:

1. Pain or burning during urination
2. Frequent urination
3. Urgency to urinate
4. Abdominal pain or discomfort
5. Bedwetting (in children who are toilet trained)

Diagnosis: The diagnosis of UTIs in children is usually based on a physical examination, a review of symptoms, and a urine analysis. In some cases, a urine culture may also be ordered to determine the specific type of bacteria causing the infection. Additional imaging tests may be ordered to evaluate the urinary tract for abnormalities or to rule out more serious conditions.

Treatment: The treatment of UTIs in children usually involves antibiotics to eliminate the infection. The specific antibiotic prescribed will depend on the age of the child, the severity of the infection, and the type of bacteria causing the infection. In some cases, hospitalization may be necessary for intravenous antibiotics or for more severe infections.

Prevention: Prevention of UTIs in children involves a few simple steps such as:

1. Encouraging good hygiene practices such as wiping front to back after bowel movements.
2. Making sure that children stay well-hydrated.
3. Encouraging children to urinate frequently, particularly after sex or bowel movements.
4. Treating any underlying conditions that increase the risk of UTIs.

UTIs are a common infection in children that can be effectively treated with antibiotics. Early diagnosis and prompt treatment can prevent complications and reduce the risk of recurrent infections.

Vesicoureteral Reflux (VUR)

Vesicoureteral reflux (VUR) is a condition that occurs when urine flows back from the bladder into the ureters and sometimes into the kidneys. It is a relatively common condition in infants and children and can be a risk factor for urinary tract infections (UTIs) and kidney damage. In this response, we will discuss VUR in the pediatric population, including its causes, symptoms, diagnosis, and treatment options.

Causes: VUR occurs when the valve between the ureter and the bladder does not function properly. This can happen because the valve is too weak or does not close tightly enough. In some cases, VUR may be caused by a blockage or abnormality in the urinary tract, such as an obstruction or a structural defect.

Symptoms: VUR may not cause any symptoms, but in some cases, it can lead to UTIs, kidney infections, and other complications. Children with VUR may experience symptoms such as:

1. Fever
2. Abdominal or back pain
3. Pain or burning during urination
4. Urinary frequency or urgency
5. Bedwetting (in children who are toilet trained)
6. High blood pressure

Diagnosis: VUR is usually diagnosed through a combination of tests, including a physical examination, urine analysis, and imaging tests. The most common imaging test used to diagnose VUR is a voiding cystourethrogram (VCUG), which involves injecting a contrast dye into the bladder and then taking X-rays to visualize the urinary tract.

Treatment: The treatment of VUR in children depends on the severity of the condition and the risk of complications. In many cases, VUR will resolve on its own as a child grows older. Some common treatment options include:

1. Antibiotics: Antibiotics may be prescribed to prevent UTIs and kidney infections while waiting for the VUR to resolve on its own.
2. Surgery: In some cases, surgery may be necessary to correct the VUR. Surgery may involve the placement of a ureteral implant or the tightening of the valve between the ureter and the bladder.
3. Observation: In mild cases of VUR, the condition may be monitored through regular follow-up appointments with a healthcare provider.

Prevention: Preventing VUR involves maintaining good urinary tract health and identifying and treating UTIs promptly. It is also important to address any underlying conditions that may increase the risk of VUR, such as blockages or structural abnormalities.

VUR is a common condition in children that can be effectively managed with appropriate treatment and monitoring. Early diagnosis and prompt treatment of VUR can help prevent complications and improve long-term outcomes for affected children.

Bedwetting

Bedwetting, also known as nocturnal enuresis, is a common condition in which a child involuntarily wets the bed during sleep. It is estimated that about 15% of children between the ages of 5 and 6 experience bedwetting, and the prevalence decreases with age. In this response, we will discuss the causes, symptoms, diagnosis, and treatment options for pediatric bedwetting.

Causes: The exact causes of bedwetting in children are not fully understood, but it is believed to be due to a combination of factors, including:

1. Delayed development of the urinary system, which can cause the child to produce more urine at night than their bladder can hold.
2. Overactive bladder muscles that cause the bladder to empty involuntarily.
3. Genetics, as bedwetting often runs in families.
4. Psychological factors, such as stress or anxiety.

Symptoms: The primary symptom of bedwetting is the involuntary release of urine during sleep. Children may also experience embarrassment or shame related to their bedwetting, which can lead to low self-esteem and social isolation.

Diagnosis: The diagnosis of bedwetting is usually based on a review of symptoms and a physical exam. In some cases, additional tests may be ordered to rule out underlying medical conditions, such as urinary tract infections, diabetes, or kidney problems.
Treatment:

There are several treatment options available for bedwetting in children, including:

1.   Behavioral therapies: Behavioral therapies, such as bladder training or positive reinforcement, can help encourage children to develop better control over their bladder and reduce the frequency of bedwetting.
2.   Medications: Medications such as desmopressin

or anticholinergics can help reduce the frequency of bedwetting by decreasing urine production or relaxing overactive bladder muscles.

3. Bedwetting alarms: Bedwetting alarms can help train children to wake up when they feel the urge to urinate, which can help them develop better bladder control over time.

4. Counseling: Counseling or therapy can help children address underlying psychological factors that may be contributing to their bedwetting.

Prevention: Preventing bedwetting involves developing good bladder habits and addressing any underlying medical or psychological conditions. Some tips for preventing bedwetting include:

1. Encouraging regular bathroom breaks during the day.
2. Limiting fluids in the evening hours.
3. Developing a consistent bedtime routine.
4. Addressing any underlying medical or psychological conditions.

Bedwetting is a common condition in children that can be effectively managed with appropriate treatment and support. Early intervention can help prevent complications and improve outcomes for affected children.

Ureteropelvic Junction Obstruction (UPJ)

Ureteropelvic junction (UPJ) obstruction is a condition in which there is a blockage or narrowing of the junction where the ureter (the tube that carries urine from the kidney to the bladder) meets the renal pelvis (the part of the kidney where urine collects). This obstruction can result in urine backing up into the kidney, leading to hydronephrosis (swelling of the kidney due to excess urine).

Causes: UPJ obstruction can be caused by a variety of factors, including:

1. Congenital abnormalities: In some cases, UPJ obstruction is present at birth due to a malformation of the ureter or renal pelvis.
2. Scarring or narrowing of the ureter: This can be caused by previous surgery or trauma, infection, or inflammation.
3. Abnormal blood vessels: An abnormal blood vessel near the UPJ can compress the ureter and cause obstruction.

Symptoms: The most common symptom of UPJ obstruction is pain in the flank or back, which can be intermittent or persistent. Other symptoms may include:

1. Blood in the urine
2. Frequent urination
3. Urinary tract infections
4. Nausea and vomiting

Diagnosis: UPJ obstruction is typically diagnosed through a combination of imaging studies and urine tests. Imaging studies such as ultrasound, CT scan, or MRI can help identify the presence of hydronephrosis and the location and severity of the obstruction. Urine tests can help identify any signs of infection or blood in the urine.
Treatment:

The treatment for UPJ obstruction depends on the severity of the obstruction and the presence of any associated complications. Mild cases may be managed with close monitoring and regular imaging studies to ensure that the obstruction does not worsen. In more severe cases, treatment options may include:

1. Surgery: In some cases, surgery may be necessary to remove the obstruction and allow urine to flow freely from the kidney to the bladder. The type of surgery

depends on the location and severity of the obstruction.

2.   Stent placement: A stent is a small tube that can be inserted into the ureter to help keep it open and allow urine to flow freely. Stents may be used as a temporary measure to relieve the obstruction until surgery can be performed, or they may be used long-term in cases where surgery is not feasible.

3.   Observation: In some cases, the obstruction may be mild enough that it does not require intervention, and the condition can be managed with regular monitoring and imaging studies.

Prevention: There are no known methods for preventing UPJ obstruction. However, prompt diagnosis and treatment can help prevent complications and improve outcomes for affected individuals.

UPJ obstruction is a condition in which there is a blockage or narrowing of the junction where the ureter meets the renal pelvis, leading to urine backing up into the kidney. Prompt diagnosis and treatment are important to prevent complications and improve outcomes for affected individuals. Treatment options depend on the severity of the obstruction and may include surgery, stent placement, or observation.

Bladder Exstrophy

Pediatric bladder exstrophy is a rare congenital anomaly that affects the development of the urinary system in infants. It occurs when the lower abdominal wall fails to develop normally during fetal development, leading to the exposure of the bladder to the outside of the body. Bladder exstrophy can occur alone or as part of a broader condition called the exstrophy-epispadias complex (EEC). In EEC, the bladder exstrophy is accompanied by abnormalities of the urethra, genitalia, and pelvis.

Symptoms: The characteristic feature of bladder exstrophy is the protrusion of the bladder through the abdominal wall, which results in the exposure of the bladder mucosa to the outside world. This exposes the bladder to various irritants, including urine, feces, and bacteria, which can lead to inflammation, infection, and damage to the bladder mucosa.

Other signs and symptoms of bladder exstrophy may include:

- An unusually small penis or an enlarged clitoris in girls
- Inwardly turned feet (clubfoot)
- A split in the pelvic bones
- Urinary incontinence
- A urinary tract infection

Causes: The exact cause of bladder exstrophy is unknown, but it is believed to result from a combination of genetic and environmental factors. The condition is thought to be due to a failure of the mesodermal tissue in the fetus to properly develop, leading to the abnormal formation of the bladder and the lower abdominal wall.

Treatment: The treatment of bladder exstrophy involves surgical repair, which aims to reconstruct the lower abdominal wall, the bladder, and the urethra. The timing and extent of the surgical repair may depend on the severity of the condition, the age of the child, and the presence of associated abnormalities.

The first surgery usually takes place within the first few days after birth and aims to close the bladder exstrophy and reconstruct the pelvic bones. Later surgeries may be needed to reconstruct the bladder and the urethra, as well as to correct any associated abnormalities.

After surgery, the child will need long-term follow-up care, which may include regular monitoring of the bladder function, the urinary tract, and the kidney function. The child may also need additional treatments, such as medications or catheterizations, to manage urinary incontinence or other urinary problems.

Bladder exstrophy is a rare congenital anomaly that affects the development of the urinary system in infants. It requires prompt and specialized surgical repair, followed by long-term follow-up care, to prevent complications and to ensure the best possible outcome for the child.

Congenital Anomalies of the Kidney and Urinary Tract

Congenital anomalies of the kidney and urinary tract (CAKUT) are a group of disorders that affect the development of the kidneys, ureters, bladder, and urethra during fetal development. These abnormalities may occur alone or as part of a broader genetic syndrome. CAKUT is a common cause of kidney disease in children and can lead to chronic kidney disease and end-stage renal disease if left untreated. Here are some common congenital anomalies of the kidney and urinary tract:

1. Renal agenesis: This is a condition where one or both kidneys fail to develop during fetal development. Renal agenesis can cause complications such as urinary tract infections, hypertension, and kidney damage.
2. Multicystic dysplastic kidney: This is a condition where one or both kidneys have multiple cysts instead of normal kidney tissue. This can cause kidney function to be impaired, but many children with this condition can live a normal life without any treatment.

3. Vesicoureteral reflux: This is a condition where urine flows backward from the bladder into the ureters, which can lead to urinary tract infections and kidney damage. Treatment options include antibiotics, surgery, or the use of a device to stop urine from flowing backward.

4. Hydronephrosis: This is a condition where urine backs up into the kidneys, causing them to become swollen. Hydronephrosis can be caused by blockages in the urinary tract or by a structural abnormality in the kidney. Treatment may involve surgery or the use of a stent to help drain the urine.

5. Obstructive uropathy: This is a condition where the flow of urine is blocked, which can cause kidney damage and lead to chronic kidney disease. Obstructive uropathy can be caused by a variety of conditions, including ureteropelvic junction obstruction, ureteral strictures, or bladder outlet obstruction.

6. Polycystic kidney disease: This is a genetic disorder where numerous cysts develop in the kidneys, causing them to become enlarged and impairing their function. Polycystic kidney disease can lead to kidney failure, and treatment options may include medications, surgery, or dialysis.

Treatment for CAKUT depends on the specific type and severity of the condition. In some cases, the condition may be treated with medication or surgery, while in other cases, the focus may be on managing symptoms and preventing complications. Children with CAKUT may require ongoing monitoring and care from a pediatric nephrologist to ensure that their kidneys are functioning properly and to prevent complications such as urinary tract infections and kidney damage.

Phimosis

Phimosis is a condition in which the foreskin of the penis is tight or constricted, making it difficult or impossible to retract the foreskin over the glans of the penis. Pediatric phimosis refers to this condition in boys who are still in their childhood and have not yet reached puberty. It is a common condition and affects approximately 10% to 20% of boys.

There are two types of phimosis: physiologic and pathologic. Physiologic phimosis is normal and occurs in all newborn boys. The foreskin is tightly adhered to the glans penis at birth and gradually separates over time. This process can take several years, and it is normal for boys to have a tight foreskin until they reach puberty. Pathologic phimosis, on the other hand, is a condition in which the foreskin is abnormally tight or constricted and cannot be retracted.

Symptoms of phimosis include difficulty retracting the foreskin, pain or discomfort during urination or sexual activity, inflammation and redness of the foreskin, and recurrent urinary tract infections.

Treatment for phimosis depends on the severity of the condition. In most cases, physiologic phimosis requires no treatment, and the foreskin will naturally separate over time. However, if the condition is causing discomfort or difficulty with urination, gentle stretching exercises and the use of a steroid cream can be helpful. In severe cases of pathologic phimosis, circumcision may be necessary.

It is important to note that circumcision is a major surgical procedure and should not be undertaken lightly. Parents should discuss the risks and benefits of circumcision with their healthcare provider before making a decision. Complications of circumcision can include bleeding, infection, and scarring.

Phimosis is a common and usually benign condition that will resolve on its own over time. However, if the condition is causing discomfort or difficulty with urination, parents should seek medical attention to determine the appropriate course of treatment.

Hypospadias

Hypospadias is a congenital condition in which the urethral opening is located on the underside of the penis instead of at the tip. It is the most common congenital anomaly affecting the male external genitalia and occurs in approximately 1 in 200 to 1 in 300 live male births. Pediatric hypospadias can range in severity from mild to severe, and the treatment options depend on the location and severity of the malformation.

Symptoms of hypospadias include a urethral opening on the underside of the penis, a downward curve of the penis during an erection, spraying of urine during urination, and difficulty with sexual intercourse in severe cases.

The exact cause of hypospadias is not fully understood, but it is thought to be due to a combination of genetic and environmental factors. It is more common in boys with a family history of the condition, as well as those born to mothers who were exposed to certain medications or chemicals during pregnancy.

Treatment for hypospadias depends on the severity and location of the malformation. Mild cases may not require treatment, while more severe cases may require surgery to correct the position of the urethral opening. Surgery may also be necessary to correct any associated penile curvature.

The most common surgical procedure for hypospadias repair

is called the tubularized incised plate (TIP) repair. In this procedure, the urethral plate is widened and then sutured to create a new urethral tube. In more severe cases, a two-stage repair may be necessary, in which the urethral plate is reconstructed in the first stage, and the new urethral tube is created in the second stage.

Complications of hypospadias surgery can include bleeding, infection, and fistula formation, which is an abnormal connection between the urethra and the skin. Long-term outcomes of surgery are generally good, with most boys achieving a normal appearance and function of the penis.

Hypospadias is a common congenital condition that requires prompt diagnosis and appropriate treatment. Treatment options depend on the severity and location of the malformation, and surgical repair is often necessary to correct the position of the urethral opening.

Inguinal Hernias

An inguinal hernia occurs when a portion of intestine or other abdominal contents protrudes through a weakened area or opening in the abdominal wall near the groin. Pediatric inguinal hernias are common, affecting approximately 1% to 5% of all infants and children. They are more common in boys than girls and are typically diagnosed within the first year of life.

Symptoms of inguinal hernias can include a bulge or swelling in the groin area that becomes more noticeable when the child is crying or straining, pain or discomfort in the groin area, and difficulty with bowel movements or urination.

The exact cause of inguinal hernias is not fully understood, but it is thought to be due to a combination of genetic and environmental factors. Certain conditions, such as premature birth and low birth weight, can also increase the risk of developing an inguinal hernia.

Treatment for inguinal hernias is surgical, and the surgery is typically performed on an outpatient basis. During the surgery, the hernia sac is identified and repaired using sutures or a mesh patch. In some cases, the surgeon may need to remove a portion of the intestine if it has become trapped or strangulated within the hernia.

Complications of inguinal hernia surgery are relatively rare but can include bleeding, infection, and recurrence of the hernia.

If left untreated, inguinal hernias can become incarcerated or strangulated, which is a medical emergency. In these cases, the blood supply to the trapped portion of intestine can become compromised, leading to tissue damage and even death.

Inguinal hernias are a common condition that requires prompt diagnosis and appropriate treatment. Surgery is the primary treatment option, and the procedure is typically performed on an outpatient basis.

Penile Adhesions and Skin Bridges

Penile adhesions and skin bridges are conditions that involve the fusion or connection of the skin on the penis, which can cause difficulty with urination, hygiene, and sexual function. These conditions are common in male infants and young boys and can be caused by a variety of factors, including poor hygiene, infection, and inflammation.

Penile adhesions occur when the foreskin becomes stuck to the glans of the penis, preventing the foreskin from retracting fully. This can cause difficulty with urination and lead to inflammation and infection. Skin bridges, on the other hand, occur when the skin on the shaft of the penis becomes attached to the glans, creating a bridge-like structure.

Symptoms of penile adhesions and skin bridges can include difficulty with urination, redness or swelling of the penis, and pain or discomfort during sexual activity.

Treatment for penile adhesions and skin bridges depends on the severity and location of the condition. In mild cases, gentle retraction of the foreskin or separation of the skin bridge may be possible using lubrication or topical steroids. In more severe cases, surgical intervention may be necessary to separate the fused skin.

Surgical treatment options for penile adhesions and skin bridges include circumcision, partial circumcision, or a dorsal slit procedure. Circumcision involves removal of the entire foreskin, while partial circumcision involves removal of only the affected area of skin. The dorsal slit procedure involves making a small incision on the top of the foreskin to relieve pressure and allow for easier retraction.

Complications of surgery for penile adhesions and skin bridges are generally rare but can include bleeding, infection, and scarring. Parents should discuss the risks and benefits of surgery with their healthcare provider to determine the best course of treatment for their child.

Prevention of penile adhesions and skin bridges involves proper hygiene and care of the penis. Parents should ensure that their child's penis is cleaned regularly, and they should avoid pulling back on the foreskin forcefully, as this can cause damage and inflammation.

Penile adhesions and skin bridges are common conditions that can cause difficulty with urination, hygiene, and sexual function. Treatment options depend on the severity and location of the condition, and surgery may be necessary in more severe cases.

Labial Adhesions

Labial adhesions, also known as labial agglutination, occur when the inner labia of the female genitalia become stuck together. This condition is most common in prepubescent girls and is thought to be caused by a combination of factors, including poor hygiene, infection, and hormonal imbalances.

Symptoms of labial adhesions can include difficulty with urination, discomfort or pain in the genital area, and recurrent urinary tract infections. In severe cases, labial adhesions can also cause difficulty with sexual function.

Treatment for labial adhesions typically involves the use of topical estrogen cream, which helps to promote the separation of the fused skin. The cream is applied to the affected area twice a day for several weeks, and gentle separation of the labia may also be necessary to ensure that the cream can reach the fused area.

In cases where topical estrogen cream is not effective, surgical intervention may be necessary to separate the labia. Surgery typically involves the use of a local anesthetic and involves making a small incision to separate the fused skin. Complications of surgery for labial adhesions are generally rare but can include bleeding, infection, and scarring.

Prevention of labial adhesions involves proper hygiene and care of the genital area. Parents should ensure that their child's genital area is cleaned regularly and thoroughly, and they should encourage their child to practice good hygiene habits as they grow older.

Labial adhesions are a common condition that can cause difficulty with urination, discomfort, and pain in the genital area, and recurrent urinary tract infections. Treatment options include the use of topical estrogen cream or surgical intervention, depending on the severity of the condition.

CHAPTER 13

Ophthalmology

Pediatric ophthalmology is a medical and surgical subspecialty that deals with eye disorders and vision problems in children. Some of the common diagnoses treated by pediatric ophthalmologists include:

1. Amblyopia (lazy eye): This is a condition where the vision in one eye does not develop properly during childhood. Treatment includes patching the good eye and vision therapy.

2. Strabismus (crossed eyes): This is a condition where the eyes do not align properly. Treatment includes eyeglasses, eye muscle exercises, or surgery.

3. Refractive errors (nearsightedness, farsightedness, and astigmatism): These are common vision problems in children that can be corrected with eyeglasses or contact lenses.

4. Congenital cataracts: These are cloudy areas in the lens of the eye that are present at birth. Treatment includes surgery to remove the cataract and restore vision.

5. Retinopathy of prematurity: This is a condition that affects premature infants and can cause abnormal blood vessel growth in the retina, leading to vision problems. Treatment includes laser therapy or surgery.

6. Ptosis (droopy eyelid): This is a condition where the upper eyelid droops over the eye. Treatment includes

surgery to lift the eyelid.

7. Eye infections: These can be caused by bacteria, viruses, or fungi and include conditions like conjunctivitis (pink eye) and keratitis. Treatment includes antibiotic or antiviral eye drops.

8. Blocked tear duct/Tearing: This can be caused by a blocked tear duct, and treatment includes massage, antibiotics, or surgery.

9. Eye injuries: These can include corneal abrasions, foreign bodies in the eye, and traumatic injuries to the eye. Treatment depends on the severity of the injury and may include antibiotics, eye patches, or surgery.

Pediatric ophthalmologists play an important role in the diagnosis and treatment of eye disorders and vision problems in children, helping to ensure that their eyesight develops properly and they achieve their full potential.

Amblyopia

Amblyopia, also known as "lazy eye," is a vision disorder that occurs in children typically before the age of eight. It occurs when the brain and the eye are not working together correctly, causing one eye to have better visual acuity than the other. The brain learns to ignore the image from the weaker eye, leading to a loss of visual acuity in that eye over time.

There are three main types of amblyopia: strabismic, refractive, and deprivation. Each type has different causes and treatments.

1. Strabismic amblyopia: This type of amblyopia occurs when one eye is misaligned or turns inward or outward. The brain receives two different images from the two eyes, and it learns to ignore the image from the misaligned eye. This can lead to a loss of visual acuity in that eye over time. Treatment usually involves correcting the

alignment of the eyes through eyeglasses, patching, or surgery.

2.	Refractive amblyopia: This type of amblyopia occurs when one eye has a significantly different refractive error (such as nearsightedness, farsightedness, or astigmatism) than the other eye. The brain learns to ignore the blurry image from the eye with the refractive error, leading to a loss of visual acuity in that eye over time. Treatment usually involves correcting the refractive error through eyeglasses, contact lenses, or refractive surgery.

3.	Deprivation amblyopia: This type of amblyopia occurs when there is a physical obstruction, such as a cataract, that prevents light from entering the eye. The brain learns to ignore the image from the obstructed eye, leading to a loss of visual acuity in that eye over time. Treatment usually involves removing the obstruction through surgery or other medical procedures.

It's important to note that the earlier amblyopia is detected and treated, the better the outcome. Children should have their vision checked regularly, and any signs of amblyopia should be addressed promptly. Treatment may involve a combination of glasses, patching, eye drops, or surgery. A comprehensive eye exam by an eye care professional is recommended for all children, starting at the age of six months.

Amblyopia is a common vision disorder in children that can be effectively treated with early intervention.

Strabismus

Strabismus, also known as "crossed eyes," is a vision disorder that occurs in children typically before the age of six. It occurs when the eyes are not aligned properly and point in different directions. One eye may turn inward, outward, upward, or downward while the other eye looks straight ahead.

There are different types of strabismus, including:

1. Esotropia: This is the most common type of strabismus in children, and it occurs when one eye turns inward towards the nose.
2. Exotropia: This occurs when one eye turns outward away from the nose.
3. Hypertropia: This occurs when one eye turns upward.
4. Hypotropia: This occurs when one eye turns downward.

The causes of strabismus in children are not fully understood, but they may include problems with the muscles that control eye movement, problems with the nerves that control the muscles, or a family history of the disorder. Strabismus can also occur as a result of other vision problems, such as nearsightedness, farsightedness, or astigmatism.

Symptoms of strabismus include:

1. Crossed or misaligned eyes.
2. Double vision.
3. Squinting or closing one eye.
4. Tilting the head to one side.
5. Poor depth perception.

Treatment of strabismus depends on the type and severity of the condition. The main goal of treatment is to realign the eyes and restore binocular vision, which allows the brain to use both eyes together. Treatment options include:

1. Eyeglasses: In some cases, eyeglasses can help correct the underlying refractive error that is causing the strabismus.
2. Patching: Patching the stronger eye can help improve vision in the weaker eye by forcing the brain to use the weaker eye more.
3. Vision therapy: This type of therapy involves exercises and activities designed to improve eye alignment and

coordination.

4. Surgery: In more severe cases, surgery may be necessary to realign the eyes. This typically involves tightening or loosening the muscles that control eye movement.

Early detection and treatment of strabismus is crucial for optimal outcomes. Children should have their eyes checked regularly, and any signs of strabismus should be addressed promptly. Treatment may involve a combination of glasses, patching, vision therapy, or surgery. A comprehensive eye exam by an eye care professional is recommended for all children, starting at the age of six months.

Strabismus is a common vision disorder in children that can be effectively treated with early intervention.

Refractive Errors

Refractive errors are common vision disorders that affect children. Refractive errors occur when the shape of the eye or the curvature of the cornea causes light to focus incorrectly on the retina, leading to blurry vision. There are four main types of refractive errors in children:

1. Myopia: Myopia, or nearsightedness, occurs when the eyeball is too long, causing light to focus in front of the retina instead of on it. This makes distant objects appear blurry, while close objects appear clear.
2. Hyperopia: Hyperopia, or farsightedness, occurs when the eyeball is too short, causing light to focus behind the retina instead of on it. This makes close objects appear blurry, while distant objects appear clear.
3. Astigmatism: Astigmatism occurs when the cornea or lens is irregularly shaped, causing light to focus on multiple points instead of a single point on the retina. This makes objects appear distorted or blurry at all distances.

4. Presbyopia: Presbyopia is an age-related condition that typically affects people over the age of 40. It occurs when the lens of the eye becomes less flexible, making it difficult to focus on close objects.

The causes of refractive errors in children are not fully understood, but they may include genetics, environmental factors, or a combination of both. Symptoms of refractive errors in children include:

1. Squinting or closing one eye.
2. Tilting the head to one side.
3. Difficulty reading or seeing the blackboard at school.
4. Headaches or eye strain.
5. Rubbing the eyes frequently.

Treatment of refractive errors in children usually involves corrective eyewear, such as glasses or contact lenses. In some cases, surgery may be necessary to correct severe refractive errors or astigmatism. It's important to note that early detection and treatment of refractive errors is crucial for optimal outcomes. Children should have their eyes checked regularly, and any signs of refractive errors should be addressed promptly. A comprehensive eye exam by an eye care professional is recommended for all children, starting at the age of six months.

Refractive errors are common vision disorders that can affect a child's ability to see clearly. Treatment typically involves corrective eyewear or, in some cases, surgery. Parents and caregivers should be aware of the signs of refractive errors and seek medical attention promptly if they suspect their child may be affected.

Congenital Cataracts

Congenital cataracts are a type of cataract that occurs in

infants and young children. Cataracts are characterized by clouding of the lens of the eye, which can cause vision loss or blindness if left untreated. Congenital cataracts are present at birth or develop shortly after, and can affect one or both eyes.

There are several causes of congenital cataracts, including genetics, infections during pregnancy, trauma, metabolic disorders, or unknown factors. Some cases may also be associated with other developmental abnormalities or syndromes.

Symptoms of congenital cataracts in infants and young children may include:

1. Poor visual acuity or low vision.
2. Nystagmus (involuntary eye movements).
3. Strabismus (misalignment of the eyes).
4. White or cloudy pupil.
5. Abnormal red reflex (an orange or white reflection seen in the pupil when light is shone into the eye).

The diagnosis of congenital cataracts is typically made through a comprehensive eye examination by an ophthalmologist. This may include a dilated eye exam, a visual acuity test, and imaging tests such as ultrasound or MRI.

Treatment for congenital cataracts usually involves surgery to remove the affected lens and replace it with an artificial intraocular lens. The timing of surgery depends on the severity of the cataract, the age of the child, and the presence of other eye conditions. In some cases, surgery may be delayed to allow the eye to mature or to address other health concerns. After surgery, the child may need to wear glasses or contact lenses to correct any residual refractive error.

Prognosis for congenital cataracts depends on several factors, including the severity and location of the cataract, the age of the child at the time of diagnosis and treatment, and the presence of other eye conditions. In general, early diagnosis and prompt treatment can improve the chances of a good visual outcome.

Congenital cataracts are a type of cataract that occurs in infants and young children. Diagnosis is made through a comprehensive eye examination, and treatment typically involves surgery to remove the affected lens and replace it with an artificial intraocular lens. Early diagnosis and prompt treatment can improve the chances of a good visual outcome.

Retinopathy of Prematurity

Retinopathy of prematurity (ROP) is a disorder that affects the eyes of premature infants. It occurs when the blood vessels that supply the retina (the part of the eye responsible for visual processing) fail to develop properly, leading to abnormal growth of blood vessels and potential vision loss.

The exact cause of ROP is not fully understood, but it is believed to be related to the immature development of the retina in premature infants. Other risk factors that can increase the likelihood of developing ROP include low birth weight, high oxygen levels, prolonged mechanical ventilation, and certain medications.

Symptoms of ROP may not be apparent initially, but can progress quickly and cause irreversible vision loss. Some signs of ROP include:

1. Abnormal blood vessel growth in the retina.
2. Poor pupil response to light.
3. Abnormal eye movements.
4. Strabismus (misaligned eyes).
5. Poor visual acuity or low vision.

Diagnosis of ROP is made through a comprehensive eye examination by an ophthalmologist who specializes in the

BRIAN WALTER TEMPLE M.D.

treatment of retinal disorders. The examination may include a dilated eye exam, retinal imaging, and other tests to assess the severity of the disease.

Treatment for ROP depends on the severity of the disease and may include:

1.   Observation: Mild cases of ROP may not require treatment and can be monitored closely by an ophthalmologist.
2.   Laser therapy: Laser therapy can be used to destroy the abnormal blood vessels in the retina and prevent further growth.
3.   Cryotherapy: Cryotherapy involves using freezing temperatures to destroy the abnormal blood vessels in the retina.
4.   Surgery: In severe cases of ROP, surgery may be necessary to repair the retina and prevent vision loss.

Prognosis for ROP depends on the severity of the disease and the promptness of treatment. Mild cases of ROP may resolve on their own without treatment, while severe cases can lead to permanent vision loss or blindness if left untreated.

Retinopathy of Prematurity is a disorder that affects the eyes of premature infants and can lead to potential vision loss if left untreated. Diagnosis is made through a comprehensive eye examination, and treatment may include observation, laser therapy, cryotherapy, or surgery. Early detection and prompt treatment are crucial for a good visual outcome.

Ptosis

Ptosis is a drooping of the upper eyelid that occurs in infants and children. It can affect one or both eyes and can be caused by a variety of factors, including congenital defects, nerve or muscle disorders, trauma, or unknown causes.

Symptoms of ptosis may include:

1. Drooping of the upper eyelid that covers part or all of the pupil.
2. Uneven appearance of the eyes.
3. Eye strain or fatigue.
4. Head tilting or chin raising to compensate for the drooping eyelid.

Diagnosis of ptosis is made through a comprehensive eye examination by an ophthalmologist. This may include a visual acuity test, a measurement of the degree of eyelid droop, and assessment of the muscle function and nerve function of the eye.

Treatment for ptosis depends on the underlying cause and severity of the condition. Mild cases of ptosis may not require treatment, while severe cases may require surgical correction to lift the drooping eyelid.

Surgical correction of ptosis is typically done under general anesthesia and involves tightening or repositioning the muscles or tendons that control eyelid movement. In some cases, a small weight may be attached to the eyelid to help it stay open. The timing of surgery depends on the severity of the ptosis and the impact it is having on the child's vision.

Prognosis for ptosis depends on the underlying cause and the success of the surgical intervention. In general, early diagnosis and prompt treatment can improve the chances of a good visual outcome.

Ptosis is a drooping of the upper eyelid that can affect one or both eyes and can be caused by a variety of factors. Diagnosis is made through a comprehensive eye examination, and treatment may include observation or surgical correction depending on the severity of the condition. Early diagnosis and prompt treatment can improve the chances of a good visual outcome.

Eye Infections

Pediatric eye infections refer to any type of infection that affects the eye or its surrounding tissues in children. There are several types of pediatric eye infections, each with their own symptoms and causes.

1. Conjunctivitis: Conjunctivitis, also known as pink eye, is a common eye infection in children caused by viruses, bacteria, or allergies. It is characterized by redness, itchiness, and discharge from the eye. Treatment depends on the underlying cause and may include eye drops, antibiotics, or antihistamines.
2. Stye: A stye is an infection of the eyelid that causes a red, painful bump to form. It is typically caused by a bacterial infection and can be treated with warm compresses and antibiotics.
3. Orbital cellulitis: Orbital cellulitis is a serious infection of the tissues surrounding the eye that can spread to the eye itself. Symptoms include swelling, pain, and redness around the eye, fever, and difficulty moving the eye. Treatment usually involves hospitalization and intravenous antibiotics.
4. Keratitis: Keratitis is an infection of the cornea, the clear outer layer of the eye. It can be caused by bacteria, viruses, fungi, or parasites and can result in blurred vision, pain, and sensitivity to light. Treatment depends on the underlying cause and may include antiviral, antibiotic, or antifungal medications.
5. Blepharitis: Blepharitis is an infection of the eyelids that causes redness, itching, and flaking of the skin around the eye. Treatment includes warm compresses and antibiotic ointments or drops.

Prevention of pediatric eye infections includes good hygiene practices, such as frequent hand washing, avoiding touching the eyes, and not sharing personal items, like towels or makeup.

Eye infections are common in children and can be caused by a variety of factors, including viruses, bacteria, fungi, and parasites. Symptoms and treatment depend on the type of infection and the underlying cause. Prevention includes good hygiene practices and avoiding contact with infected individuals. It is important to seek medical attention promptly if a child exhibits any symptoms of a pediatric eye infection to prevent potential complications.

Blocked Tear Ducts and Tearing

Blocked tear ducts and tearing in pediatric patients are common conditions that can cause discomfort and affect the quality of life of infants and young children.

Blocked tear ducts occur when there is an obstruction in the tear ducts, which are the tiny tubes that drain tears from the eyes into the nose. This can cause the tears to overflow onto the cheeks, leading to excessive tearing, crusty eyes, and possible infections. The most common cause of blocked tear ducts in infants is the failure of the nasolacrimal duct to fully develop at birth. In some cases, blockages can also be caused by inflammation or injury.

Treatment for blocked tear ducts in infants typically involves massaging the tear ducts several times a day to help open them up. Antibiotic eye drops or ointments may also be prescribed to prevent infections. In some cases, a procedure called probing and irrigation may be necessary to clear the blockage. This involves inserting a thin probe into the tear duct and irrigating it with saline solution to remove any obstruction.

Excessive tearing in pediatric patients can also be caused by other conditions, such as allergies, eye infections, or foreign objects in the eye. It can also be a symptom of a more serious condition, such as glaucoma or a tumor.

Treatment for excessive tearing in pediatric patients depends on the underlying cause. If the cause is an infection, antibiotics may be prescribed. If the cause is an allergy, antihistamines may be used to reduce symptoms. In some cases, surgery may be necessary to correct structural abnormalities or remove tumors.

Blocked tear ducts and excessive tearing are common conditions in pediatric patients that can be caused by a variety of factors. Treatment depends on the underlying cause and may include massaging the tear ducts, antibiotics, antihistamines, or surgery.

Pediatric Eye Injuries

Pediatric eye injuries are a common occurrence and can range from minor injuries such as corneal abrasions to more serious injuries such as orbital fractures or globe rupture. These injuries can result from various causes including accidents, falls, sports injuries, and physical abuse. It is important to seek medical attention promptly if a child exhibits symptoms of an eye injury to prevent potential complications.

Some common types of pediatric eye injuries include:

1. Corneal Abrasions: A corneal abrasion occurs when the surface of the cornea, the clear front part of the eye, is scratched or scraped. Symptoms may include eye pain, redness, and sensitivity to light. Treatment typically

involves antibiotics and lubricating eye drops.
2.   Chemical Burns: Chemical burns can occur when chemicals come into contact with the eye. This can lead to severe eye pain, vision loss, and even blindness. Treatment involves flushing the eye with water or saline and seeking immediate medical attention.
3.   Orbital Fractures: Orbital fractures occur when one or more bones surrounding the eye are broken. Symptoms may include swelling, bruising, and a change in vision. Treatment typically involves surgery to repair the fracture.
4.   Globe Rupture: A globe rupture occurs when the outer layer of the eye is torn, which can result in loss of vision or even blindness. This is a medical emergency that requires immediate treatment and surgery.
5.   Penetrating Eye Injury: A penetrating eye injury occurs when an object penetrates the eye, such as a sharp object or a projectile. This is also a medical emergency that requires immediate treatment and surgery.

Prevention of eye injuries includes wearing protective eyewear during sports and other activities, using age-appropriate toys, and keeping hazardous materials out of reach of children. It is also important to teach children about the potential risks and how to avoid them.

Eye injuries can range from minor injuries such as corneal abrasions to more serious injuries such as orbital fractures or globe rupture. Treatment depends on the type and severity of the injury and may include antibiotics, surgery, or other interventions. Prevention includes using protective eyewear and teaching children about potential risks.

CHAPTER 14

Genetics

Pediatric genetic doctors, also known as pediatric geneticists, diagnose and manage genetic conditions in children. Some of the common diagnoses treated by pediatric genetic doctors include:

1. Down syndrome: This is a genetic disorder caused by an extra copy of chromosome 21. Children with Down syndrome may have developmental delays, intellectual disability, and physical features such as a flattened face and small stature.

2. Cystic fibrosis: This is a genetic disorder that affects the lungs, pancreas, and other organs. Children with cystic fibrosis may have difficulty breathing, frequent lung infections, and digestive problems.

3. Sickle cell disease: This is an inherited blood disorder that affects the shape of red blood cells. Children with sickle cell disease may have chronic pain, an increased risk of infections, and other complications.

4. Muscular dystrophy: This is a group of genetic disorders that cause progressive muscle weakness and degeneration. Children with muscular dystrophy may have difficulty walking, breathing, and performing daily activities.

5. Neurofibromatosis: This is a genetic disorder that causes tumors to grow on nerves throughout the body. Children

with neurofibromatosis may have skin abnormalities, vision problems, and other complications.

6. Fragile X syndrome: This is a genetic disorder that causes intellectual disability and behavioral problems. Children with Fragile X syndrome may have delayed speech and language development, social anxiety, and other symptoms.

7. Turner syndrome: This is a genetic disorder that affects only females and is caused by missing or incomplete X chromosomes. Children with Turner syndrome may have short stature, delayed puberty, and other physical and developmental abnormalities.

8. Inherited metabolic disorders: These are genetic disorders that affect the body's ability to break down and use nutrients. Children with inherited metabolic disorders may have problems with growth and development, as well as neurological and other complications.

Genetic doctors work closely with families to diagnose and manage genetic conditions in children, helping to improve outcomes and quality of life for affected children and their families.

Down Syndrome

Down syndrome is a genetic disorder that occurs when there is an extra copy of chromosome 21. This results in certain physical and intellectual characteristics and can lead to a variety of health concerns. Down syndrome is the most common chromosomal disorder, affecting approximately 1 in every 700 births worldwide.

Physical Characteristics: Individuals with Down syndrome typically have distinct physical characteristics, including:

1. Small stature

2. Short neck
3. Flat facial profile
4. Upward slanting eyes
5. Small ears
6. Protruding tongue
7. Low muscle tone

Intellectual and Behavioral Characteristics: Individuals with Down syndrome may also have intellectual and behavioral characteristics, including:

1. Mild to moderate intellectual disability
2. Delayed speech and language development
3. Learning difficulties
4. Impulsivity
5. Hyperactivity
6. Social and emotional difficulties

Health Concerns: Individuals with Down syndrome are also at increased risk for certain health concerns, including:

1. Congenital heart defects
2. Respiratory infections
3. Hearing loss
4. Vision problems
5. Thyroid problems
6. Digestive problems
7. Leukemia
8. Alzheimer's disease

Treatment and Management:

While there is no cure for Down syndrome, treatment and management can help individuals with the condition to lead fulfilling lives. Treatment may include speech therapy, physical therapy, occupational therapy, and educational programs tailored to the individual's needs. Management of health concerns may include regular medical check-ups, medications, and surgery if necessary.

Support for individuals with Down syndrome and their families is also important. There are various support groups and organizations that can provide resources, information, and community for those affected by the condition.

Cystic Fibrosis

Cystic fibrosis (CF) is a genetic disorder that primarily affects the respiratory, digestive, and reproductive systems. It is caused by mutations in the CFTR gene, which encodes for a protein that regulates the movement of salt and water in and out of cells. This results in the production of thick, sticky mucus in the affected organs.

Symptoms: CF symptoms vary widely from person to person and can include:

1. Persistent coughing
2. Shortness of breath
3. Wheezing
4. Recurrent lung infections
5. Digestive problems, such as malnutrition, poor growth, and difficulty absorbing nutrients
6. Infertility in males due to blocked or absent vas deferens
7. Delayed puberty
8. Nasal polyps
9. Clubbing of the fingers and toes

Diagnosis: CF can be diagnosed through various tests, including sweat tests, genetic testing, and lung function tests. Sweat tests measure the amount of salt in sweat, which is typically elevated in individuals with CF. Genetic testing can identify mutations in the CFTR gene, while lung function tests measure the amount of air that can be exhaled from the lungs.

Treatment: While there is no cure for CF, treatment can help manage symptoms and improve quality of life. Treatment options may include:

1. Airway clearance techniques, such as chest physiotherapy and nebulized medications, to help clear mucus from the lungs.
2. Antibiotics to treat and prevent lung infections.
3. Pancreatic enzyme supplements to aid in digestion.
4. Nutritional supplements to ensure adequate nutrient intake.
5. Lung transplant in severe cases.

Prognosis: The prognosis for CF has improved significantly in recent years, thanks to advances in treatment and management. However, the life expectancy for individuals with CF remains lower than that of the general population, with an average life expectancy of around 40 years.

Prevention: CF is an inherited disorder, so prevention involves genetic counseling for individuals and families at risk of having a child with CF. Prenatal testing is also available to identify the presence of CF in the developing fetus.

Cystic fibrosis is a genetic disorder that affects the respiratory, digestive, and reproductive systems. Symptoms vary widely, but treatment options are available to manage symptoms and improve quality of life. Prevention involves genetic counseling and prenatal testing for individuals and families at risk of having a child with CF.

Sickle Cell Anemia

Sickle cell anemia is a genetic blood disorder characterized by abnormally shaped red blood cells. This condition is caused by mutations in the HBB gene that produces hemoglobin, the protein responsible for carrying oxygen throughout the body.

In sickle cell anemia, the abnormal hemoglobin causes red blood cells to become stiff and crescent-shaped, leading to a variety of symptoms and complications.

Symptoms: Symptoms of sickle cell anemia can vary from person to person and can include:

1. Pain crises: episodes of severe pain that can last for hours to days.
2. Anemia: a shortage of red blood cells, which can cause fatigue, weakness, and shortness of breath.
3. Jaundice: yellowing of the skin and eyes due to the breakdown of red blood cells.
4. Delayed growth and development in children.
5. Increased risk of infections.
6. Vision problems, such as blurred vision and loss of vision.
7. Stroke.
8. Acute chest syndrome: a serious complication that can cause chest pain, shortness of breath, and fever.

Diagnosis: Sickle cell anemia is typically diagnosed through a blood test that checks for the presence of abnormal hemoglobin. Other tests may be done to evaluate organ function, such as a kidney function test or a lung function test.

Treatment: Treatment for sickle cell anemia aims to manage symptoms and prevent complications. Options may include:

1. Pain management: with medications and other therapies, such as heat or massage.
2. Blood transfusions: to replace damaged red blood cells and improve oxygen delivery.
3. Hydroxyurea: a medication that can increase the production of fetal hemoglobin, a type of hemoglobin that is less likely to cause sickling.
4. Bone marrow transplant: a procedure that can replace damaged bone marrow with healthy marrow from a donor.

5. Antibiotics and vaccinations: to prevent infections.
6. Education and counseling: to help manage the emotional and psychological impact of the condition.

Prognosis: The prognosis for sickle cell anemia can vary depending on the severity of the condition and the individual's overall health. With proper management and care, many individuals with sickle cell anemia are able to live active and fulfilling lives. However, the condition can be life-threatening in some cases, and individuals with sickle cell anemia may be at increased risk for certain health concerns, such as stroke, lung disease, and kidney disease.

Prevention: Sickle cell anemia is an inherited disorder, so prevention involves genetic counseling and testing for individuals and families at risk of having a child with the condition. Prenatal testing is also available to identify the presence of sickle cell anemia in the developing fetus.

Sickle cell anemia is a genetic blood disorder characterized by abnormally shaped red blood cells. Symptoms can vary widely and may include pain crises, anemia, and increased risk of infections. Treatment options are available to manage symptoms and prevent complications, and prevention involves genetic counseling and testing.

Muscular Dystrophy

Muscular dystrophy (MD) is a group of genetic disorders that cause progressive muscle weakness and degeneration. The most common form of MD is Duchenne muscular dystrophy, which primarily affects boys and is caused by mutations in the DMD gene.

Symptoms: The symptoms of MD can vary depending on the type and severity of the condition. Common symptoms may include:

1.   Muscle weakness, particularly in the hips, pelvis, thighs, and shoulders.
2.   Difficulty with walking, running, and climbing stairs.
3.   Muscle wasting and degeneration.
4.   Contractures, or joint stiffness and immobility.
5.   Cardiac and respiratory problems.
6.   Difficulty with speech, chewing, and swallowing.
7.   Learning disabilities.

Diagnosis: MD is typically diagnosed through a combination of physical examinations, genetic testing, and diagnostic tests such as electromyography (EMG) and muscle biopsy. Early diagnosis is important for effective management and treatment.

Treatment: While there is no cure for MD, treatment options are available to manage symptoms and improve quality of life. These may include:

1.   Physical therapy: to maintain muscle strength and flexibility.
2.   Occupational therapy: to improve daily living skills and adapt to mobility challenges.
3.   Mobility aids: such as braces, wheelchairs, and scooters.
4.   Medications: to manage symptoms such as pain, inflammation, and muscle spasms.
5.   Breathing assistance: such as noninvasive ventilation or tracheostomy.
6.   Cardiac care: to monitor and manage heart function.
7.   Clinical trials: to test new treatments and therapies.

Prognosis: The prognosis for MD can vary depending on the type and severity of the condition. Some forms of MD progress slowly and may not significantly impact life expectancy, while others can be life-threatening and may reduce lifespan. Early diagnosis and management can improve outcomes and quality of life.

Prevention: As MD is a genetic disorder, prevention involves genetic counseling and testing for individuals and families at risk of having a child with the condition. Prenatal testing is also available to identify the presence of MD in the developing fetus.

Muscular Dystrophy is a group of genetic disorders that cause progressive muscle weakness and degeneration. Symptoms can vary widely and may include muscle weakness, wasting, and contractures, as well as cardiac and respiratory problems. While there is no cure, treatment options are available to manage symptoms and improve quality of life. Prevention involves genetic counseling and testing.

Neurofibromatosis

Neurofibromatosis is a genetic disorder that causes the growth of benign tumors on or under the skin, along with nerve tissue. There are three types of neurofibromatosis: type 1 (NF1), type 2 (NF2), and schwannomatosis.

Symptoms: The symptoms of neurofibromatosis can vary depending on the type and severity of the condition. Common symptoms may include:

1. Skin changes: the development of small, noncancerous bumps on or under the skin.
2. Freckling: the appearance of numerous brown spots on the skin.
3. Nerve-related problems: such as numbness, tingling, weakness, and pain.
4. Vision and hearing problems: particularly in NF2, which can cause tumors to form on the nerves that control hearing and balance.
5. Bone deformities: particularly in NF1, which can cause curvature of the spine and other skeletal abnormalities.
6. Learning disabilities and cognitive impairment:

particularly in NF1, which can cause learning disabilities, attention deficits, and behavioral problems.

Diagnosis: Neurofibromatosis is typically diagnosed through a combination of physical examinations, genetic testing, and diagnostic imaging such as MRI or CT scans. Early diagnosis is important for effective management and treatment.

Treatment: While there is no cure for neurofibromatosis, treatment options are available to manage symptoms and improve quality of life. These may include:

1. Surgery: to remove tumors that are causing pain or affecting organ function.
2. Radiation therapy: to shrink tumors and alleviate symptoms.
3. Chemotherapy: to shrink tumors and slow their growth.
4. Physical therapy: to maintain muscle strength and flexibility.
5. Mobility aids: such as braces, wheelchairs, and scooters.
6. Medications: to manage symptoms such as pain, inflammation, and seizures.
7. Clinical trials: to test new treatments and therapies.

Prognosis: The prognosis for neurofibromatosis can vary depending on the type and severity of the condition. Some forms of neurofibromatosis progress slowly and may not significantly impact life expectancy, while others can be life-threatening and may reduce lifespan. Early diagnosis and management can improve outcomes and quality of life.

Prevention: As neurofibromatosis is a genetic disorder, prevention involves genetic counseling and testing for individuals and families at risk of having a child with the condition. Prenatal testing is also available to identify the presence of neurofibromatosis in the developing fetus.

Neurofibromatosis is a genetic disorder that causes the

growth of benign tumors on or under the skin, along with nerve tissue. Symptoms can vary widely and may include skin changes, nerve-related problems, vision and hearing problems, bone deformities, and learning disabilities. While there is no cure, treatment options are available to manage symptoms and improve quality of life. Prevention involves genetic counseling and testing.

Fragile X-Syndrome

Fragile X syndrome is a genetic disorder that affects the development of the brain and other parts of the body. It is caused by a mutation on the FMR1 gene, which provides instructions for making a protein called fragile X mental retardation protein (FMRP). Without enough FMRP, the brain does not develop properly, leading to intellectual and developmental disabilities.

Symptoms: The symptoms of fragile X syndrome can vary widely depending on the individual and the severity of the condition. Some common symptoms may include:

1. Intellectual disability: ranging from mild to severe.
2. Developmental delays: particularly in language and social skills.
3. Behavioral problems: such as hyperactivity, anxiety, aggression, and autism-like behaviors.
4. Physical features: such as a long and narrow face, large ears, and a prominent forehead.
5. Connective tissue problems: such as flat feet, a high-arched palate, and joint problems.
6. Sensory processing issues: such as hypersensitivity to sound and touch.

Diagnosis: Fragile X syndrome is typically diagnosed through genetic testing, which can detect the FMR1 gene mutation. Prenatal testing is also available for families at risk of having a child with fragile X syndrome.

Treatment: There is no cure for fragile X syndrome, but there are treatment options available to manage symptoms and improve quality of life. These may include:

1. Educational and behavioral interventions: such as speech therapy, occupational therapy, and behavioral therapy to address learning and developmental delays and behavior problems.
2. Medications: such as stimulants to treat hyperactivity, and antidepressants to manage anxiety and aggression.
3. Assistive technology: such as communication devices and adaptive equipment to support mobility and independence.
4. Clinical trials: to test new treatments and therapies.

Prognosis: The prognosis for fragile X syndrome can vary widely depending on the severity of the condition and the individual's response to treatment. With early intervention and ongoing support, many individuals with fragile X syndrome are able to lead fulfilling lives and achieve a degree of independence. However, some may require lifelong assistance and support.

Prevention: As fragile X syndrome is a genetic disorder, prevention involves genetic counseling and testing for individuals and families at risk of having a child with the condition. Prenatal testing is also available to identify the presence of fragile X syndrome in the developing fetus.

Fragile X syndrome is a genetic disorder that affects the development of the brain and other parts of the body. Symptoms can vary widely and may include intellectual and developmental disabilities, behavioral problems, physical features, and sensory processing issues. While there is no cure, treatment options are available to manage symptoms and improve quality of life. Prevention involves genetic counseling and testing.

Turner Syndrome

Turner syndrome, also known as monosomy X, is a genetic condition that affects females. It occurs when a female has only one X chromosome or is missing a portion of one of the X chromosomes. Turner syndrome can cause a variety of physical and developmental issues.

Symptoms: The symptoms of Turner syndrome can vary widely, but may include:

1. Short stature: Girls with Turner syndrome are typically shorter than average, with a height of less than 5 feet.
2. Delayed puberty: Girls with Turner syndrome may not undergo puberty at the same time as their peers.
3. Infertility: Many girls and women with Turner syndrome are unable to conceive naturally.
4. Heart and kidney problems: Some individuals with Turner syndrome may have heart or kidney abnormalities.
5. Learning difficulties: Girls with Turner syndrome may have difficulty with math, spatial skills, and memory.
6. Social and emotional issues: Girls with Turner syndrome may have difficulty with social skills and making friends.

Diagnosis: Turner syndrome is usually diagnosed during childhood or adolescence. A doctor may suspect Turner syndrome if a girl has short stature, delayed puberty, or other physical abnormalities. A blood test can confirm the diagnosis by detecting the absence of one X chromosome or a partial deletion of the chromosome.

Treatment: There is no cure for Turner syndrome, but there

are treatments available to manage symptoms and improve quality of life. These may include:

1. Growth hormone therapy: This treatment can increase height and improve bone density.
2. Estrogen replacement therapy: This treatment can induce puberty and prevent osteoporosis.
3. Fertility treatments: Some women with Turner syndrome may be able to conceive with the help of fertility treatments such as in vitro fertilization.
4. Surgery: Surgery may be needed to correct heart or kidney abnormalities.
5. Educational and behavioral interventions: These may be needed to address learning difficulties and social and emotional issues.

Prognosis: The prognosis for Turner syndrome can vary widely depending on the severity of the condition and the individual's response to treatment. With early intervention and ongoing support, many individuals with Turner syndrome are able to lead fulfilling lives and achieve a degree of independence. However, some may require lifelong assistance and support.

Prevention: As Turner syndrome is a genetic disorder, prevention involves genetic counseling and testing for individuals and families at risk of having a child with the condition. Prenatal testing is also available to identify the presence of Turner syndrome in the developing fetus.

Turner syndrome is a genetic condition that affects females and can cause a variety of physical and developmental issues. Diagnosis is usually made during childhood or adolescence. While there is no cure, treatment options are available to manage symptoms and improve quality of life. Prevention involves genetic counseling and testing.

Inherited Metabolic Disorders

Inherited metabolic disorders (IMDs) are a group of genetic disorders that affect the body's metabolism, the process of breaking down food and converting it into energy and other substances that the body needs to function. These disorders result from defects in the enzymes and proteins involved in metabolism, leading to an abnormal buildup or deficiency of certain substances in the body.

There are more than 500 known IMDs, and they can affect people of all ages and ethnicities. They are often classified according to the type of substance that is affected, such as amino acids, carbohydrates, or fats.

Symptoms: The symptoms of IMDs can vary widely depending on the specific disorder and the severity of the condition. Some common symptoms include:

1. Failure to thrive: Infants and young children with IMDs may have poor growth and development.
2. Developmental delays: Children with IMDs may experience delays in reaching developmental milestones such as walking and talking.
3. Intellectual disability: Some IMDs can cause intellectual disability or learning difficulties.
4. Seizures: Some IMDs can cause seizures or other neurological problems.
5. Organ dysfunction: Some IMDs can affect the function of organs such as the liver, kidneys, and heart.
6. Abnormal physical features: Some IMDs can cause physical features such as facial abnormalities or skeletal deformities.

Diagnosis: Diagnosis of IMDs typically involves a combination of physical examination, medical history, and laboratory tests. These tests may include blood tests, urine tests, and genetic testing to identify the specific metabolic disorder and determine its severity.

Treatment: Treatment for IMDs varies depending on the specific disorder and the severity of the condition. Some treatment options may include:

1. Dietary changes: Some IMDs can be managed through dietary changes, such as avoiding certain foods or taking supplements.
2. Medications: Some IMDs may be treated with medications that can help manage symptoms and prevent complications.
3. Enzyme replacement therapy: Some IMDs can be treated with enzyme replacement therapy, which involves replacing the deficient enzyme with a synthetic version.
4. Gene therapy: In some cases, gene therapy may be used to correct the genetic defect that causes the IMD.
5. Organ transplantation: In severe cases, organ transplantation may be necessary to replace a damaged organ.

Prognosis: The prognosis for IMDs varies widely depending on the specific disorder and the severity of the condition. Some IMDs can be managed with dietary changes and medications, while others may require more aggressive treatments such as enzyme replacement therapy or organ transplantation. Some IMDs can be life-threatening if left untreated.

Prevention: As IMDs are genetic disorders, prevention involves genetic counseling and testing for individuals and families at risk of having a child with an IMD. Prenatal testing is also available to identify the presence of an IMD in the developing fetus.

Inherited metabolic disorders are a group of genetic disorders that affect the body's metabolism, leading to an abnormal buildup or deficiency of certain substances in the body. Diagnosis involves physical examination, medical history, and laboratory tests, and treatment options vary depending on the specific disorder and severity of the condition. Prevention involves genetic counseling and testing.

CHAPTER 15

Otolaryngology

Pediatric otolaryngology, also known as pediatric ENT (ear, nose, and throat) is a specialized field of medicine that focuses on the diagnosis and treatment of disorders related to the head and neck in children. This field deals with a wide range of issues that affect children, from common conditions such as ear infections to more complex conditions such as congenital anomalies.

Pediatric otolaryngologists are trained to provide medical and surgical care to children with conditions that affect the ear, nose, throat, and related structures of the head and neck. These specialists work in collaboration with other healthcare professionals, including pediatricians, audiologists, speech-language pathologists, and other specialists as needed to provide comprehensive care for children.

Conditions Treated in Pediatric Otolaryngology:

1. Ear disorders: Pediatric otolaryngologists treat a wide range of ear disorders, including ear infections, hearing loss, tinnitus, and vertigo.
2. Nose disorders: This includes treatment of conditions such as allergies, sinusitis, deviated septum, and nasal

polyps.

3.   Throat disorders: Common throat conditions treated by pediatric otolaryngologists include tonsillitis, adenoiditis, hoarseness, and voice disorders.

4.   Airway disorders: Pediatric otolaryngologists also treat airway disorders such as cleft palate, tracheostomy, and laryngomalacia.

5.   Head and neck tumors: This includes the treatment of benign and malignant tumors of the head and neck.

6.   Craniofacial anomalies: This includes the treatment of congenital disorders such as cleft lip and palate, hemangiomas, and vascular malformations.

Ear Disorders

Ear disorders refer to a range of conditions that affect the ear and hearing in children. These disorders can occur in one or both ears and can be congenital or acquired. In this article, we will discuss the most common pediatric ear disorders, their causes, symptoms, diagnosis, and treatment.

Otitis Media:

1.   Otitis media is a common pediatric ear disorder characterized by inflammation or infection of the middle ear. The most common cause of otitis media is a bacterial or viral infection that spreads from the upper respiratory tract. Symptoms may include ear pain, fever, irritability, hearing loss, and drainage from the ear. Diagnosis is made by a physical examination of the ear, and treatment may include antibiotics, pain relief medications, or the placement of tympanostomy tubes to drain the fluid.

Otitis Externa:

2.   Otitis externa, also known as swimmer's ear, is an infection or inflammation of the external ear canal. It is

caused by a bacterial or fungal infection or irritation of the ear canal due to excess moisture or foreign objects. Symptoms may include ear pain, itching, redness, and drainage from the ear. Diagnosis is made by a physical examination of the ear, and treatment may include antibiotics, ear drops, and pain relief medications.

Congenital Hearing Loss:

3. Congenital hearing loss is a hearing impairment that is present at birth or acquired shortly after. It may be caused by genetic factors, infections during pregnancy, or other factors that affect the development of the ear. Symptoms may include delayed speech and language development, difficulty hearing, and lack of response to sounds. Diagnosis is made through hearing screening tests, and treatment may include hearing aids, cochlear implants, or other interventions depending on the severity of the hearing loss.

Tympanic Membrane Perforation:

4. Tympanic membrane perforation is a hole or tear in the eardrum. It can be caused by injury to the ear, infection, or pressure changes due to altitude changes. Symptoms may include ear pain, hearing loss, and discharge from the ear. Diagnosis is made by a physical examination of the ear, and treatment may include antibiotics, ear drops, or surgery to repair the eardrum.

Cholesteatoma:

5. Cholesteatoma is a rare but serious pediatric ear disorder characterized by the growth of abnormal skin cells in the middle ear. It may be caused by repeated ear infections or a congenital defect. Symptoms may include ear pain, hearing loss, and drainage from the ear. Diagnosis is

made by a physical examination of the ear and imaging tests, and treatment may include antibiotics or surgery to remove the abnormal skin cells and repair the damage.

Tinnitus:

6.   Tinnitus is a ringing, buzzing, or other noise in the ear that is not caused by an external source. It may be caused by exposure to loud noise, ear infections, or other factors. Symptoms may include hearing a constant sound in the ear, difficulty sleeping, and difficulty concentrating. Diagnosis is made through a hearing evaluation, and treatment may include medication, therapy, or sound therapy to manage the symptoms.

Ear disorders in the pediatric population can significantly impact a child's quality of life, and early diagnosis and treatment are crucial. Treatment may include medication, ear drops, surgery, or hearing aids, depending on the specific disorder and severity of symptoms. It is important for parents to be aware of the signs and symptoms of pediatric ear disorders and seek medical attention promptly if they suspect their child has an ear problem.

Nose Disorders

Disorders to the nose refer to a range of conditions that affect the nasal passages and sinuses in children. These disorders can range from minor problems such as nasal congestion to more severe conditions such as nasal polyps or tumors. In this article, we will discuss the most common pediatric nose disorders, their causes, symptoms, diagnosis, and treatment.

Nasal Congestion:

1.   Nasal congestion is a common nose disorder in children characterized by the inflammation of the nasal passages. It can be caused by a viral infection,

allergies, or exposure to irritants such as cigarette smoke. Symptoms may include difficulty breathing, runny nose, and sneezing. Treatment may include saline nasal sprays, decongestants, or antihistamines.

Allergic Rhinitis:

2.   Allergic rhinitis is a condition caused by an allergic reaction to substances such as pollen, dust, or animal dander. It is a common nose disorder in children and can be seasonal or year-round. Symptoms may include nasal congestion, runny nose, sneezing, and itchy eyes. Treatment may include antihistamines, nasal corticosteroids, or immunotherapy.

Nasal Polyps:

3.   Nasal polyps are non-cancerous growths that develop in the lining of the nose or sinuses. They can be caused by chronic inflammation due to conditions such as allergic rhinitis or cystic fibrosis. Symptoms may include nasal congestion, runny nose, and difficulty breathing. Treatment may include medication, such as corticosteroids or surgery to remove the polyps.

Deviated Septum:

4.   A deviated septum occurs when the nasal septum, the cartilage that separates the two nostrils, is crooked or misaligned. It can be a congenital condition or result from injury. Symptoms may include nasal congestion, difficulty breathing, and frequent nosebleeds. Treatment may include medication or surgery to correct the alignment of the septum.

Sinusitis:

5.   Sinusitis is a condition characterized by inflammation

or infection of the sinuses, which are air-filled cavities behind the nasal passages. It can be caused by a bacterial or viral infection, allergies, or exposure to irritants. Symptoms may include nasal congestion, headache, facial pain, and fever. Treatment may include antibiotics, nasal corticosteroids, or sinus surgery.

Choanal Atresia:

6.   Choanal atresia is a congenital disorder characterized by a blockage of the nasal passages. It occurs when the membrane that separates the nasal passages from the mouth fails to break down during fetal development. Symptoms may include difficulty breathing, nasal congestion, and feeding difficulties. Treatment may include surgery to open the blocked nasal passage.

Disorders of the nose can significantly impact a child's quality of life, and early diagnosis and treatment are crucial. Treatment may include medication, surgery, or immunotherapy, depending on the specific disorder and severity of symptoms. It is important for parents to be aware of the signs and symptoms of pediatric nose disorders and seek medical attention promptly if they suspect their child has a nose problem.

Throat Disorders

Throat disorders refer to a range of conditions that affect the throat or pharynx in children. These disorders can range from minor problems such as sore throat to more severe conditions such as tonsillitis or throat cancer. In this article, we will discuss the most common pediatric throat disorders, their causes, symptoms, diagnosis, and treatment.

Sore Throat:

1.   Sore throat is a common throat disorder in children

characterized by pain, irritation, or itchiness in the throat. It can be caused by a viral or bacterial infection, allergies, or exposure to irritants such as cigarette smoke. Symptoms may include difficulty swallowing, fever, and swollen lymph nodes. Treatment may include pain relievers, rest, and hydration.

Tonsillitis:

2. Tonsillitis is a condition caused by inflammation or infection of the tonsils, which are the two lymph nodes at the back of the throat. It can be caused by a viral or bacterial infection, and symptoms may include sore throat, fever, and swollen tonsils. Treatment may include antibiotics, pain relievers, or in severe cases, tonsillectomy.

Pharyngitis:

3. Pharyngitis is a condition caused by inflammation or infection of the pharynx, which is the part of the throat behind the mouth and nasal cavity. It can be caused by a viral or bacterial infection, allergies, or exposure to irritants such as cigarette smoke. Symptoms may include sore throat, fever, and swollen lymph nodes. Treatment may include antibiotics, pain relievers, and rest.

Laryngitis:

4. Laryngitis is a condition caused by inflammation or infection of the larynx or voice box. It can be caused by a viral or bacterial infection, overuse of the voice, or exposure to irritants such as cigarette smoke. Symptoms may include hoarseness, difficulty speaking, and sore throat. Treatment may include rest, hydration, and voice therapy.

Vocal Cord Nodules:

5.   Vocal cord nodules are growths that develop on the vocal cords due to overuse or misuse of the voice. They are common in children who use their voices excessively, such as singers or cheerleaders. Symptoms may include hoarseness, difficulty speaking, and pain when speaking or singing. Treatment may include voice therapy or surgery to remove the nodules.

Epiglottitis:

6.   Epiglottitis is a rare but serious condition caused by inflammation or infection of the epiglottis, which is a flap of tissue that covers the trachea during swallowing. It can be caused by a bacterial infection, and symptoms may include difficulty swallowing, drooling, and high fever. Treatment may include hospitalization, antibiotics, and intubation in severe cases.

Throat disorders can significantly impact a child's quality of life, and early diagnosis and treatment are crucial. Treatment may include medication, surgery, or voice therapy, depending on the specific disorder and severity of symptoms. It is important for parents to be aware of the signs and symptoms of pediatric throat disorders and seek medical attention promptly if they suspect their child has a throat problem.

Airway Disorders

Pediatric airway disorders refer to a group of conditions that affect the airways in children, including the trachea, bronchi, and lungs. These conditions can range from mild to life-threatening and can cause symptoms such as difficulty breathing, coughing, and wheezing. In this article, we will discuss the most common pediatric airway disorders, their causes, symptoms, diagnosis, and treatment.

Asthma:

1.　　Asthma is a chronic lung disease that causes inflammation and narrowing of the airways, making it difficult to breathe. It is a common pediatric airway disorder that can be triggered by allergens, irritants, or exercise. Symptoms may include wheezing, coughing, and shortness of breath. Treatment may include bronchodilators, corticosteroids, and avoidance of triggers.

Bronchitis:

2.　Bronchitis is an inflammation of the bronchial tubes, which are the air passages that lead to the lungs. It is a common pediatric airway disorder that can be caused by viral or bacterial infections. Symptoms may include coughing, wheezing, and difficulty breathing. Treatment may include rest, hydration, and medication such as bronchodilators and corticosteroids.

Croup:

3.　　Croup is a viral infection that affects the upper airways, including the larynx and trachea. It is a common pediatric airway disorder that causes a barking cough, hoarseness, and difficulty breathing. Treatment may include humidified air, corticosteroids, and epinephrine.

Epiglottitis:

4.　Epiglottitis is a rare but serious infection that affects the epiglottis, which is a flap of tissue that covers the trachea during swallowing. It is a pediatric airway disorder that can cause difficulty breathing, drooling, and high fever. Treatment may include hospitalization, antibiotics, and intubation in severe cases.

Foreign Body Aspiration:

5.   Foreign body aspiration occurs when a child inhales a foreign object into the airways. It is a pediatric airway disorder that can cause coughing, wheezing, and difficulty breathing. Treatment may include removal of the object through bronchoscopy.

Laryngomalacia:

6.   Laryngomalacia is a congenital airway disorder that affects the larynx, causing it to collapse during inspiration. It is a pediatric airway disorder that can cause stridor, or high-pitched breathing, and difficulty feeding. Treatment may include observation, weight management, or surgery in severe cases.

Tracheomalacia:

7.   Tracheomalacia is a congenital or acquired airway disorder that affects the trachea, causing it to collapse during breathing. It is a pediatric airway disorder that can cause wheezing, coughing, and difficulty breathing. Treatment may include observation, weight management, or surgery in severe cases.

Pediatric airway disorders can significantly impact a child's quality of life and require prompt diagnosis and treatment. Treatment may include medication, humidified air, or surgery, depending on the specific disorder and severity of symptoms.

Head and Neck Tumors

Pediatric head and neck tumors are growths that develop

in the tissues of the head and neck in children. They can be benign (non-cancerous) or malignant (cancerous), and can affect different areas such as the thyroid gland, salivary glands, and lymph nodes. In this article, we will discuss the most common pediatric head and neck tumors, their causes, symptoms, diagnosis, and treatment.

Lymphoma:

1. Lymphoma is a type of cancer that affects the lymphatic system, which is part of the immune system. It can occur in the lymph nodes, tonsils, and other tissues of the head and neck. Symptoms may include swelling, pain, and fever. Treatment may include chemotherapy, radiation therapy, and surgery.

Thyroid tumors:

2. Thyroid tumors are growths that develop in the thyroid gland, which is located in the neck. They can be benign or malignant and can cause symptoms such as neck swelling, difficulty swallowing, and hoarseness. Treatment may include surgery, radiation therapy, and chemotherapy.

Salivary gland tumors:

3. Salivary gland tumors are growths that develop in the glands that produce saliva in the mouth and neck. They can be benign or malignant and can cause symptoms such as swelling, pain, and difficulty swallowing. Treatment may include surgery, radiation therapy, and chemotherapy.

Neuroblastoma:

4.   Neuroblastoma is a type of cancer that affects the nervous system and can occur in the head and neck region. It can cause symptoms such as neck swelling, pain, and difficulty swallowing. Treatment may include chemotherapy, radiation therapy, and surgery.

Rhabdomyosarcoma:

5.   Rhabdomyosarcoma is a type of cancer that affects the soft tissues of the head and neck, such as the muscles and connective tissues. It can cause symptoms such as swelling, pain, and difficulty swallowing. Treatment may include chemotherapy, radiation therapy, and surgery.

Hemangioma:

6.   Hemangioma is a benign tumor that develops in the blood vessels of the head and neck. It can cause symptoms such as swelling and redness. Treatment may include observation, medication, and surgery in severe cases.

Diagnosis of pediatric head and neck tumors may include a physical examination, imaging tests such as CT scan and MRI, and biopsy. Treatment options depend on the type of tumor, its location, and the stage of the disease. Treatment may include surgery, radiation therapy, chemotherapy, and targeted therapy. In some cases, a combination of treatments may be used.

Head and neck tumors can be a serious health concern for children. It is important for parents to be aware of the signs and symptoms of these tumors and seek medical attention promptly if they suspect their child may have a head or neck tumor. Early diagnosis and treatment can improve outcomes and increase the chances of successful treatment.

Craniofacial Anomalies

Craniofacial anomalies refer to a group of conditions that affect the development of the head and face in children. These conditions can affect the skull, the bones of the face, and the tissues and structures of the mouth and throat. Craniofacial anomalies can range from mild to severe and can cause physical and functional impairments, as well as emotional and social challenges. In this article, we will discuss some of the most common pediatric craniofacial anomalies, their causes, symptoms, diagnosis, and treatment.

Cleft lip and palate:

1.   Cleft lip and palate are birth defects that occur when the tissues that form the lips and mouth do not fuse properly during fetal development. This can result in an opening in the lip or roof of the mouth that can cause feeding difficulties, speech problems, and dental issues. Treatment may include surgery, dental appliances, and speech therapy.

Craniosynostosis:

2.   Craniosynostosis is a condition in which the sutures (joints) between the bones of the skull close too early, which can cause abnormal head shape and pressure on the brain. Symptoms may include an abnormally shaped head, developmental delays, and vision problems. Treatment may include surgery to correct the skull shape and relieve pressure on the brain.

Apert syndrome:

3.   Apert syndrome is a genetic condition that affects the development of the skull and face. It can cause abnormalities such as a fused skull, wide-set eyes, and

abnormal growth of the fingers and toes. Symptoms may include respiratory problems, feeding difficulties, and developmental delays. Treatment may include surgery, speech therapy, and physical therapy.

Treacher Collins syndrome:

4.   Treacher Collins syndrome is a genetic condition that affects the development of the bones and tissues of the face. It can cause abnormalities such as small or absent cheekbones, underdeveloped jaws, and abnormally shaped ears. Symptoms may include hearing loss, vision problems, and difficulty breathing. Treatment may include surgery, speech therapy, and hearing aids.

Pierre Robin sequence:

5.   Pierre Robin sequence is a condition in which the lower jaw is smaller than normal, which can cause the tongue to fall back and obstruct the airway. This can result in breathing difficulties and feeding problems. Treatment may include positioning devices, feeding tubes, and surgery to correct the jaw and airway.

Diagnosis of craniofacial anomalies may involve a physical examination, medical imaging tests such as CT scans and MRI, genetic testing, and evaluation by a team of specialists such as pediatricians, geneticists, and craniofacial surgeons. Treatment may include surgical correction, orthodontic treatment, speech therapy, and other supportive therapies.

Pediatric craniofacial anomalies can have significant impacts on a child's physical, functional, and social well-being. Early diagnosis and intervention by a multidisciplinary team of specialists can improve outcomes and quality of life for affected children and their families.

CHAPTER 16

Allergy & Immunology

Pediatric allergy and immunology is a specialized field of medicine that focuses on the diagnosis and treatment of allergies and immune system disorders in children. Allergies occur when the immune system reacts to a normally harmless substance, such as pollen or food, and triggers a reaction. Immune system disorders occur when the immune system fails to function properly and can lead to infections or autoimmune diseases.

- Common medical conditions treated by pediatric allergy and immunology specialists include:
- Asthma: Asthma is a chronic respiratory condition characterized by wheezing, coughing, and difficulty breathing. Allergies are a common trigger for asthma, and pediatric allergy and immunology specialists can help identify and manage these triggers.
- Allergic rhinitis: Allergic rhinitis, also known as hay fever, is a condition that causes inflammation and irritation of the nasal passages due to allergens such as pollen, dust, or pet dander.
- Food allergies: Food allergies occur when the immune system reacts to a specific food, such as peanuts or milk, and triggers an allergic reaction. Pediatric allergy and immunology specialists can help identify and manage

food allergies.

- Eczema: Eczema, also known as atopic dermatitis, is a chronic skin condition characterized by dry, itchy, and inflamed skin. It can be triggered by allergens, and pediatric allergy and immunology specialists can help identify and manage these triggers.
- Immunodeficiency disorders: Immunodeficiency disorders are conditions in which the immune system is unable to function properly, making children more susceptible to infections. Pediatric allergy and immunology specialists can help diagnose and manage these disorders.
- Hives: Hives, also known as urticaria, are red, itchy bumps on the skin that can appear suddenly and disappear just as quickly. They are often caused by an allergic reaction to food, medication, or insect bites.
- Anaphylaxis: Anaphylaxis is a severe and potentially life-threatening allergic reaction that requires immediate medical attention. It can be triggered by food, medication, or insect bites.
- Pediatric allergy and immunology specialists use a variety of diagnostic tools to identify allergies and immune system disorders, including skin testing, blood tests, and imaging studies. Treatment options may include medications, allergy shots, and lifestyle modifications to avoid triggers.

Pediatric allergy and immunology plays an important role in the diagnosis, treatment, and management of allergies and immune system disorders in children, helping to improve their quality of life and prevent serious complications.

Asthma

Asthma is a chronic respiratory condition that affects children and is characterized by airway inflammation and hyperresponsiveness, which causes recurring episodes of wheezing, coughing, chest tightness, and shortness of breath.

Symptoms: The symptoms of pediatric asthma may include:

1. Wheezing: a whistling sound when breathing out.
2. Shortness of breath: difficulty breathing or feeling like you can't catch your breath.
3. Coughing: a persistent or recurring cough, especially at night or early in the morning.
4. Chest tightness: a feeling of tightness or pressure in the chest.
5. Rapid breathing: breathing faster than normal.

Causes: The exact causes of pediatric asthma are not fully understood, but several factors are believed to play a role, including:

1. Genetics: asthma tends to run in families.
2. Environmental factors: exposure to pollution, allergens, and respiratory infections can trigger asthma symptoms.
3. Immune system factors: some children may have an overactive immune system that triggers asthma symptoms in response to certain triggers.
4. Physical activity: physical activity can trigger asthma symptoms in some children.

Diagnosis: The diagnosis of asthma involves a combination of medical history, physical examination, and lung function tests. The medical history will involve asking questions about the child's symptoms, family history, and exposure to potential triggers. The physical examination will involve listening to the child's lungs for wheezing and other signs of respiratory distress. Lung function tests may be used to measure the child's lung function and determine the severity of the asthma.

Treatment: The goal of treatment for asthma is to control

BRIAN WALTER TEMPLE M.D.

symptoms, prevent exacerbations, and maintain normal lung function. Treatment options may include:

1. Inhaled bronchodilators: medications that relax the muscles around the airways, making it easier to breathe.
2. Inhaled corticosteroids: medications that reduce airway inflammation and prevent asthma symptoms.
3. Combination inhalers: medications that contain both a bronchodilator and a corticosteroid.
4. Oral medications: medications that can be taken orally to control asthma symptoms.
5. Immunotherapy: a treatment that involves gradually exposing the child to small amounts of an allergen to reduce their sensitivity to the allergen over time.
6. Education: teaching children and their families about asthma triggers, medications, and self-management strategies can help them better manage their symptoms.

Prevention: Preventing asthma symptoms involves identifying and avoiding triggers that can trigger asthma attacks. Some common triggers include:

1. Allergens: such as dust mites, pet dander, mold, and pollen.
2. Respiratory infections: such as colds, flu, and sinus infections.
3. Irritants: such as cigarette smoke, air pollution, and strong odors.
4. Physical activity: some children may experience asthma symptoms during or after physical activity.

Asthma is a chronic respiratory condition that affects children and is characterized by airway inflammation and hyperresponsiveness. The diagnosis involves a combination of medical history, physical examination, and lung function tests. Treatment options include medications, immunotherapy, and education. Preventing asthma symptoms involves identifying and avoiding triggers. With proper management, most children with asthma can lead healthy, active lives.

Allergic Rhinitis

Allergic rhinitis, also known as hay fever, is a common condition in pediatric patients that is caused by an allergic reaction to certain substances, such as pollen, dust mites, animal dander, and mold.
Symptoms:

The symptoms of allergic rhinitis in pediatric patients may include:

1. Sneezing: repeated sneezing or sneezing attacks.
2. Runny nose: nasal congestion and discharge that may be clear or colored.
3. Itchy nose: an itchy or tingling sensation in the nose.
4. Nasal congestion: a feeling of fullness or pressure in the nose.
5. Itchy eyes: red, watery, and itchy eyes.
6. Postnasal drip: mucus that drips down the back of the throat.
7. Fatigue: feeling tired or lethargic due to the impact of the condition on the body.

Causes: Allergic rhinitis is caused by an allergic reaction to certain substances, known as allergens. These allergens can vary depending on the season, location, and individual patient, but some of the most common allergens include:

1. Pollen: from trees, grass, and weeds.
2. Dust mites: microscopic organisms found in household dust.
3. Animal dander: skin flakes and hair from cats, dogs, and other animals.

4.   Mold: found in damp areas such as basements and bathrooms.

Diagnosis: The diagnosis of allergic rhinitis involves a combination of medical history, physical examination, and allergy testing. The medical history will involve asking questions about the child's symptoms, family history, and exposure to potential allergens. The physical examination will involve examining the child's nose, throat, and ears for signs of inflammation or other abnormalities. Allergy testing may be used to identify the specific allergens that are triggering the child's symptoms.

Treatment: The goal of treatment for allergic rhinitis is to control symptoms, prevent exacerbations, and improve the child's quality of life. Treatment options may include:

1.   Antihistamines: medications that block the release of histamine, a chemical that causes allergy symptoms.
2.   Nasal corticosteroids: medications that reduce inflammation in the nasal passages.
3.   Decongestants: medications that reduce nasal congestion.
4.   Immunotherapy: a treatment that involves gradually exposing the child to small amounts of an allergen to reduce their sensitivity to the allergen over time.
5.   Education: teaching children and their families about allergen avoidance, medications, and self-management strategies can help them better manage their symptoms.

Prevention: Preventing allergic rhinitis symptoms involves identifying and avoiding triggers that can trigger allergic reactions. Some common triggers include:

1.   Allergens: such as pollen, dust mites, animal dander, and mold.
2.   Irritants: such as cigarette smoke, air pollution, and

strong odors.

3. Physical activity: some children may experience allergic rhinitis symptoms during or after physical activity.
4. Weather changes: some children may experience symptoms during certain weather conditions.

Allergic rhinitis is a common condition in pediatric patients that is caused by an allergic reaction to certain substances, such as pollen, dust mites, animal dander, and mold. The diagnosis involves a combination of medical history, physical examination, and allergy testing. Treatment options include medications, immunotherapy, and education. Preventing allergic rhinitis symptoms involves identifying and avoiding triggers. With proper management, most children with allergic rhinitis can lead healthy, active lives.

Food Allergies

Food allergies are a common problem in pediatric patients that can cause a range of symptoms, from mild itching and swelling to severe, life-threatening reactions. Food allergies occur when the immune system overreacts to a particular food, treating it as a harmful substance.

Symptoms: The symptoms of food allergies in pediatric patients can vary depending on the severity of the reaction and the food allergen involved. Common symptoms may include:

1. Skin reactions: hives, itching, and swelling.
2. Digestive problems: abdominal pain, diarrhea, and vomiting.
3. Respiratory symptoms: coughing, wheezing, and difficulty breathing.
4. Anaphylaxis: a severe, life-threatening reaction that can cause a sudden drop in blood pressure, rapid pulse, and

loss of consciousness.

Causes: Food allergies are caused by an overreaction of the immune system to a particular food or food component. The most common food allergens in pediatric patients include:

1. Peanuts: one of the most common food allergens, which can cause severe reactions.
2. Tree nuts: such as walnuts, almonds, and cashews.
3. Milk: a common allergen in young children.
4. Eggs: another common allergen in young children.
5. Wheat: a common allergen that can cause digestive problems.
6. Soy: a common allergen that can cause skin reactions and digestive problems.
7. Fish and shellfish: common allergens that can cause severe reactions.

Diagnosis: The diagnosis of food allergies in pediatric patients involves a combination of medical history, physical examination, and allergy testing. The medical history will involve asking questions about the child's symptoms, family history of allergies, and exposure to potential allergens. The physical examination will involve examining the child for signs of allergic reactions, such as hives or swelling. Allergy testing may include skin tests or blood tests to identify the specific food allergens that are causing the child's symptoms.
Treatment:

The treatment of food allergies in pediatric patients involves avoiding the allergen that causes the reaction. This may involve reading food labels carefully and avoiding foods that contain the allergen. In severe cases, the child may need to carry an epinephrine auto-injector, which can be used to quickly treat anaphylaxis. Other treatment options may include antihistamines or corticosteroids to reduce symptoms.

Prevention: Preventing food allergies in pediatric patients involves avoiding exposure to potential allergens, especially in children who are at high risk of developing food allergies. Breastfeeding for the first six months of life may help reduce the risk of food allergies, and introducing solid foods one at a time may help identify potential allergens. In some cases, early introduction of potential allergens under medical supervision may also help reduce the risk of food allergies.

Food allergies are a common problem in pediatric patients that can cause a range of symptoms, from mild itching and swelling to severe, life-threatening reactions. The diagnosis involves a combination of medical history, physical examination, and allergy testing. Treatment options include avoiding the allergen, carrying an epinephrine auto-injector, and medications to reduce symptoms. Preventing food allergies involves avoiding exposure to potential allergens and introducing solid foods one at a time. With proper management and prevention, most children with food allergies can lead healthy, active lives.

Eczema

Eczema, also known as atopic dermatitis, is a common skin condition that affects many pediatric patients. It is a chronic inflammatory condition characterized by dry, itchy, and red patches of skin that can appear anywhere on the body.

Causes: The exact cause of eczema in pediatric patients is not known, but it is believed to be a combination of genetic and environmental factors. Children with a family history of eczema, allergies, or asthma are more likely to develop eczema. Other factors that can trigger or worsen eczema symptoms include irritants, such as soaps, detergents, and fragrances, and allergens, such as pollen and pet dander.

Symptoms: The symptoms of eczema in pediatric patients can

vary, but the most common symptoms include:

1. Dry, scaly, or cracked skin
2. Red or inflamed skin
3. Itching, which can be severe
4. Small bumps that may ooze or crust over
5. Thickened or leathery skin in areas that have been scratched repeatedly
6. Discoloration of the skin, which can be light or dark
7. Swelling or puffiness in affected areas

Diagnosis: The diagnosis of eczema in pediatric patients is based on the child's medical history and physical examination. The doctor will ask questions about the child's symptoms, including when they started and what seems to trigger them. The doctor may also perform a skin test to rule out other conditions, such as allergies or infections.

Treatment: The treatment of eczema in pediatric patients involves a combination of skin care, medication, and lifestyle changes. Skin care measures may include:

1. Using mild, fragrance-free soaps and moisturizers
2. Avoiding harsh chemicals and irritants
3. Taking short, lukewarm baths or showers
4. Using a humidifier to add moisture to the air

Medications used to treat eczema may include:

1. Topical corticosteroids to reduce inflammation and itching
2. Topical calcineurin inhibitors to reduce inflammation and itching
3. Antihistamines to reduce itching
4. Antibiotics or antifungal medications to treat infections

Lifestyle changes that can help manage eczema symptoms

may include:

1. Avoiding scratching or rubbing the affected areas
2. Wearing soft, breathable clothing
3. Identifying and avoiding triggers, such as certain foods or environmental allergens
4. Managing stress, as stress can trigger eczema symptoms

Prevention: Preventing eczema in pediatric patients can be challenging, but there are some measures that may help reduce the risk of developing eczema or worsening symptoms, such as:

1. Breastfeeding for the first six months of life, if possible
2. Avoiding exposure to tobacco smoke
3. Using fragrance-free, hypoallergenic detergents and soaps
4. Avoiding harsh chemicals and irritants, such as solvents and cleaning products
5. Identifying and avoiding triggers, such as certain foods or environmental allergens

Eczema is a common skin condition that affects many pediatric patients. It is a chronic inflammatory condition characterized by dry, itchy, and red patches of skin that can appear anywhere on the body. The treatment of eczema involves a combination of skin care, medication, and lifestyle changes. Preventing eczema in pediatric patients may involve avoiding triggers, such as certain foods or environmental allergens. With proper management and prevention, most children with eczema can lead healthy, active lives.

Pediatric Immunodeficiencies

Pediatric immunodeficiencies refer to a group of disorders characterized by a compromised or absent immune system in children. This can lead to an increased risk of infections, poor growth, and developmental delays. There are two main types of pediatric immunodeficiencies: primary immunodeficiencies and secondary immunodeficiencies.

Primary immunodeficiencies are caused by genetic defects that affect the immune system. These are usually inherited and present at birth. Some examples of primary immunodeficiencies include:

1. Severe Combined Immunodeficiency (SCID): This is a rare disorder where the child is born with little or no immune system. Children with SCID are extremely susceptible to infections and often require a bone marrow transplant.
2. Common Variable Immunodeficiency (CVID): CVID is a disorder where the immune system does not produce enough antibodies to fight infections. This leads to recurrent infections and can cause damage to organs such as the lungs and digestive system.
3. X-Linked Agammaglobulinemia (XLA): XLA is a rare disorder that affects only males. It is caused by a genetic defect that prevents the body from producing normal levels of antibodies. This leads to recurrent infections, particularly in the ears, sinuses, and lungs.

Secondary immunodeficiencies are acquired after birth and can be caused by a variety of factors, including infections, medications, and cancer treatments. Examples of secondary immunodeficiencies include:

1. HIV/AIDS: HIV attacks and destroys the immune system, leaving the child vulnerable to a range of infections and illnesses.
2. Chemotherapy and radiation therapy: These treatments can damage the immune system, leaving the child susceptible to infections.
3. Chronic illnesses such as diabetes, kidney disease, and liver disease can also compromise the immune system,

making it harder for the child to fight off infections.

The symptoms of pediatric immunodeficiencies vary depending on the type and severity of the disorder. However, some common symptoms include:

- Recurrent infections such as ear infections, sinus infections, pneumonia, and skin infections
- Failure to thrive and poor growth
- Delayed development and milestones
- Chronic diarrhea or other digestive problems
- Skin rashes or infections
- Chronic or frequent colds and flu-like symptoms

Treatment for pediatric immunodeficiencies depends on the type and severity of the disorder. Treatment options may include:

- Antibiotics and other medications to treat infections
- Immunoglobulin replacement therapy to replace missing antibodies
- Bone marrow or stem cell transplant for severe cases of primary immunodeficiencies
- Antiretroviral therapy for children with HIV/AIDS

Children with immunodeficiencies benefit from proper medical care and should take steps to prevent infections, such as practicing good hygiene and avoiding contact with sick individuals

Hives

Hives, also known as urticaria, are a common skin condition that can occur in pediatric populations. They appear as raised, red or pink welts on the skin that can be itchy and may vary in size and shape. Hives can be acute or chronic and can occur in response to a variety of triggers.

Acute hives typically last for a few hours or days and are often caused by an allergic reaction to food, medication, insect bites, or environmental factors such as pollen or animal dander. In some cases, acute hives may be caused by an infection, such as a viral or bacterial infection.

Chronic hives, on the other hand, last for more than six weeks and are often more difficult to diagnose and treat. Chronic hives can be caused by a variety of factors, including autoimmune disorders, chronic infections, and hormonal imbalances.

The symptoms of hives in pediatric populations can vary depending on the severity of the condition. Common symptoms include:

- Raised, red or pink welts on the skin
- Itching or a burning sensation
- Swelling or tightness in the throat or other areas of the body
- Difficulty breathing or swallowing
- Nausea or vomiting

In most cases, hives can be diagnosed based on a physical examination and medical history. Blood tests or skin tests may be recommended to identify the trigger of the hives, particularly in cases of chronic hives.

Treatment for hives in pediatric populations typically involves identifying and avoiding the trigger of the hives, if possible. Medications such as antihistamines may be prescribed to relieve itching and reduce swelling. In more severe cases, oral corticosteroids may be prescribed to reduce inflammation.

Preventing hives in pediatric populations involves avoiding known triggers and practicing good hygiene. This includes avoiding known allergens, such as certain foods or insect bites, and washing hands regularly to prevent the spread of infection. In cases of chronic hives, it may be necessary to make lifestyle changes, such as reducing stress and avoiding certain medications or environmental factors.

Anaphylaxis

Anaphylaxis is a serious and potentially life-threatening allergic reaction that can occur in pediatric populations. It is a medical emergency that requires prompt treatment to prevent complications and death.

Anaphylaxis can be caused by a variety of triggers, including food allergies, insect bites or stings, medication allergies, and exposure to certain environmental factors, such as latex or pollen. The symptoms of anaphylaxis can develop rapidly and may include:

- Swelling of the lips, tongue, and throat
- Difficulty breathing or wheezing
- Rapid or weak pulse
- Dizziness or fainting
- Hives or a rash
- Abdominal pain, nausea, or vomiting

If anaphylaxis is suspected, emergency medical services should be contacted immediately, and the person should be given an injection of epinephrine, which can help to open airways and increase blood pressure. Other treatments may include administration of oxygen, intravenous fluids, and medications to reduce swelling and inflammation.

Preventing anaphylaxis in pediatric populations involves identifying and avoiding known triggers, and carrying emergency medication such as epinephrine auto-injectors. Children with known allergies should wear medical alert bracelets or necklaces, and parents and caregivers should be trained to recognize the symptoms of anaphylaxis and respond quickly in case of an emergency.

CHAPTER 17

Pathology

P athology is a specialized field of medicine that focuses on the diagnosis of diseases and conditions that affect children from infancy to adolescence. Pediatric pathologists play a critical role in pediatric medicine by providing accurate and timely diagnoses that inform treatment decisions and improve outcomes for pediatric patients.

Pediatric pathologists use a variety of techniques to analyze tissue and body fluid samples, including microscopic examination, molecular and genetic analysis, and advanced imaging techniques. They work closely with other healthcare professionals, including pediatricians, pediatric surgeons, and pediatric oncologists, to provide comprehensive care for pediatric patients.

Pediatric pathologists diagnose a wide range of diseases and conditions, including:

1. Childhood cancers: Pediatric pathologists play a critical role in the diagnosis and management of childhood cancers, such as leukemia, lymphoma, and brain tumors. They use advanced laboratory techniques to analyze tissue samples and provide accurate diagnoses that inform treatment decisions.

2. Congenital abnormalities: Pediatric pathologists can

diagnose congenital abnormalities, such as heart defects, cleft lip and palate, and neural tube defects, using imaging studies and genetic testing.

3.   Infections: Pediatric pathologists can identify infectious agents, such as bacteria, viruses, and fungi, in tissue and body fluid samples using microbiological and molecular techniques.

4.   Autoimmune diseases: Pediatric pathologists can diagnose autoimmune diseases, such as juvenile rheumatoid arthritis and lupus, using laboratory tests that detect specific antibodies and other immune system markers.

5.   Metabolic disorders: Pediatric pathologists can diagnose metabolic disorders, such as phenylketonuria and cystic fibrosis, using laboratory tests that measure specific enzymes and other metabolic markers.

6.   Autopsy:

In addition to diagnosis, pediatric pathologists also play a crucial role in research and education. They conduct research to better understand the underlying mechanisms of pediatric diseases and develop new diagnostic and treatment approaches. They also provide education and training to other healthcare professionals, including medical students, residents, and fellows, to help improve the quality of care for pediatric patients.

Pediatric pathology is an essential component of pediatric medicine, providing critical diagnostic and research services that help improve the health and well-being of children.

Cancer

Pathologists play a crucial role in the diagnosis and treatment of childhood cancers. They are responsible for examining tissue samples taken from the affected area to determine the type and extent of the cancer. The pathologist's role is crucial because a correct diagnosis is essential for the selection of the most effective treatment plan.

In addition to providing an accurate diagnosis, pathologists also play a key role in determining the stage of cancer. The stage of cancer refers to the extent to which it has spread throughout the body. This information is essential for determining the appropriate course of treatment.

Pathologists also play an important role in determining the prognosis for children with cancer. The prognosis is the predicted outcome of the disease based on various factors, including the stage of cancer, the child's age, and overall health. This information can help healthcare providers and families make informed decisions about the child's care and treatment options.

Pathologists work closely with other healthcare providers, including pediatric oncologists, to develop a comprehensive treatment plan. The treatment plan typically includes a combination of surgery, radiation therapy, chemotherapy, and other supportive therapies. The pathologist's role is critical in determining the effectiveness of these treatments by monitoring the progression of cancer through follow-up biopsies and imaging studies.

Finally, pathologists play a crucial role in research efforts to improve the diagnosis and treatment of childhood cancers. They work with other researchers to develop new diagnostic tests, treatments, and therapies. By studying the molecular and genetic makeup of cancer cells, pathologists can help identify new treatment targets and develop more effective therapies.

Pathologists play an essential role in the diagnosis, staging, and treatment of childhood cancers. They work closely with other healthcare providers to develop comprehensive treatment plans and monitor the effectiveness of treatment.

Pathologists also play a critical role in research efforts to improve the diagnosis and treatment of childhood cancers.

Congenital Abnormalities

Pathologists play an important role in the diagnosis and management of congenital abnormalities in children. Congenital abnormalities are structural or functional abnormalities present at birth and can involve various organs and body systems.

Pathologists play a crucial role in the diagnosis of congenital abnormalities by examining tissue samples obtained through biopsies, autopsies, and other diagnostic procedures. They analyze the samples and use their expertise to identify any structural or functional abnormalities that may be present. This information is essential for accurately diagnosing the condition and guiding the course of treatment.

Pathologists can also help to determine the cause of the congenital abnormality, which may be genetic, environmental, or a combination of both. By analyzing the tissue samples, pathologists can identify genetic mutations, chromosomal abnormalities, or other factors that may have contributed to the development of the abnormality.

In addition to diagnosis, pathologists also play a key role in developing treatment plans for children with congenital abnormalities. They work closely with other healthcare providers, such as pediatricians and surgeons, to develop comprehensive treatment plans that address the specific needs of the child.

Pathologists also play a critical role in ongoing research efforts aimed at improving the diagnosis and treatment of congenital abnormalities. By studying the genetic and molecular mechanisms underlying these conditions, pathologists can help identify new targets for treatment and develop more effective therapies.

Finally, pathologists are also involved in counseling and support services for families of children with congenital abnormalities. They can provide information about the condition, treatment options, and potential outcomes, as well as offer emotional support and guidance throughout the diagnosis and treatment process.

In summary, pathologists play an essential role in the diagnosis, management, and research of congenital abnormalities in children. They are instrumental in accurately diagnosing the condition, determining the cause, developing treatment plans, and providing counseling and support services to families.

Pediatric Infections

Pathologists play a critical role in the diagnosis and management of pediatric infections. Pathology is the study of disease, and pathologists are physicians who specialize in the study of disease through examination of tissues, cells, and bodily fluids. They use their expertise to identify the causes of diseases and help determine the appropriate treatment and management.

In the case of pediatric infections, pathologists can be involved in several ways:

1. Diagnosis: Pathologists play a key role in the diagnosis of infectious diseases by examining specimens obtained from infected children, such as blood, urine, stool, or tissue samples. They use various laboratory techniques, such as culture, serology, molecular testing, and histopathology, to identify the infectious agent responsible for the disease.

2. Prognosis: Pathologists can also help predict the course and outcome of infectious diseases by analyzing the severity and extent of tissue damage caused by the infection. For example, in cases of viral infections, pathologists can examine tissue samples to determine the extent of damage to organs such as the liver, lung, or brain, which can help guide treatment decisions.

3. Treatment: Pathologists can provide valuable information to guide the selection and monitoring of antimicrobial therapy. For example, they can perform susceptibility testing to determine which antibiotics are most effective against the infectious agent causing the disease. Pathologists can also monitor the response to treatment by examining specimens obtained during treatment to assess whether the infectious agent has been eradicated.

4. Outbreak investigation: In cases of outbreaks of infectious diseases in pediatric populations, pathologists can play a crucial role in identifying the source and mode of transmission of the infection. They can examine specimens from infected children and compare them to specimens from other patients to determine whether they are caused by the same infectious agent.

Pathologists are essential members of the healthcare team in the management of pediatric infections. Their expertise in the diagnosis, prognosis, and treatment of infectious diseases can help ensure that infected children receive appropriate and timely care, leading to better outcomes.

Autoimmune Disorders

Pathologists play an important role in the diagnosis

and management of autoimmune disorders. Autoimmune disorders are conditions in which the immune system mistakenly attacks the body's own tissues, resulting in inflammation and tissue damage. Pathology is the study of disease, and pathologists are physicians who specialize in the study of disease through examination of tissues, cells, and bodily fluids. They use their expertise to identify the causes of diseases and help determine the appropriate treatment and management.

In the case of autoimmune disorders, pathologists can be involved in several ways:

1. Diagnosis: Pathologists play a key role in the diagnosis of autoimmune disorders by examining tissues or bodily fluids obtained from affected patients. They use various laboratory techniques, such as immunohistochemistry and flow cytometry, to identify the presence of autoantibodies and immune cells that are characteristic of autoimmune diseases. For example, in patients with lupus, pathologists can examine kidney biopsy samples to identify the presence of immune deposits, which can help confirm the diagnosis.

2. Prognosis: Pathologists can help predict the course and outcome of autoimmune disorders by analyzing the severity and extent of tissue damage caused by the immune system. For example, in patients with rheumatoid arthritis, pathologists can examine joint tissues to assess the extent of inflammation and damage, which can help guide treatment decisions.

3. Treatment: Pathologists can provide valuable information to guide the selection and monitoring of treatment for autoimmune disorders. For example, they can perform tests to determine the effectiveness of immunosuppressive therapies, such as corticosteroids or biologic agents. Pathologists can also monitor the

response to treatment by examining tissues or bodily fluids obtained during treatment to assess whether the inflammation and tissue damage have been reduced.

4. Research: Pathologists are involved in ongoing research to better understand the causes and mechanisms of autoimmune disorders. By studying tissues and bodily fluids obtained from affected patients, pathologists can identify new biomarkers and potential targets for therapy.

Pathologists are essential members of the healthcare team in the diagnosis and management of autoimmune disorders. Their expertise in the identification of characteristic immune cells and antibodies, as well as the assessment of tissue damage, can help ensure that patients receive appropriate and timely care, leading to better outcomes.

Metabolic Disorders

Pathologists play a crucial role in the diagnosis and management of metabolic disorders. Metabolic disorders are genetic conditions that affect the body's ability to convert food into energy, resulting in the accumulation of toxic substances and the malfunction of organs and tissues. Pathology is the study of disease, and pathologists are physicians who specialize in the study of disease through the examination of tissues, cells, and bodily fluids. They use their expertise to identify the causes of diseases and help determine the appropriate treatment and management.

In the case of metabolic disorders, pathologists can be involved in several ways:

1. Diagnosis: Pathologists play a key role in the diagnosis of metabolic disorders by examining tissues or bodily fluids obtained from affected patients. They use various laboratory techniques, such as histology,

immunohistochemistry, and molecular testing, to identify the presence of specific metabolic abnormalities. For example, in patients with lysosomal storage disorders, pathologists can examine tissues such as liver or spleen biopsy samples to identify the accumulation of specific enzymes, which can help confirm the diagnosis.

2. Prognosis: Pathologists can help predict the course and outcome of metabolic disorders by analyzing the extent of organ damage caused by metabolic abnormalities. For example, in patients with mitochondrial disorders, pathologists can examine muscle biopsy samples to assess the extent of mitochondrial dysfunction, which can help guide treatment decisions.

3. Treatment: Pathologists can provide valuable information to guide the selection and monitoring of treatment for metabolic disorders. For example, they can perform tests to determine the effectiveness of enzyme replacement therapies or other interventions. Pathologists can also monitor the response to treatment by examining tissues or bodily fluids obtained during treatment to assess whether the metabolic abnormalities have been corrected.

4. Research: Pathologists are involved in ongoing research to better understand the causes and mechanisms of metabolic disorders. By studying tissues and bodily fluids obtained from affected patients, pathologists can identify new biomarkers and potential targets for therapy.

Pathologists are essential members of the healthcare team in the diagnosis and management of metabolic disorders. Their expertise in the identification of specific metabolic abnormalities and the assessment of tissue damage can help ensure that patients receive appropriate and timely care, leading to better outcomes.

Autopsy

A pediatric autopsy is a medical examination of the body of a deceased child to determine the cause of death. Autopsies are performed by forensic pathologists who specialize in examining the human body to determine the cause and manner of death.

The primary objective of a pediatric autopsy is to determine the cause of death accurately. This information is essential for determining the child's medical history, identifying possible genetic or environmental factors that may have contributed to the death, and providing information that can help prevent similar deaths in the future.

The pediatric autopsy procedure typically involves the following steps:

1. Consent: The parents or legal guardians of the child must give consent for the autopsy to be performed. The decision to proceed with an autopsy can be challenging for families, so it is important that the process is thoroughly explained to them.
2. External Examination: The body of the child is thoroughly examined externally to document any injuries or abnormalities. The child's height, weight, and other physical characteristics are also recorded.
3. Internal Examination: The body is opened, and the internal organs are examined. Samples of tissue are taken for further analysis. The pathologist examines the organs to determine the cause of death, and any other underlying medical conditions that may have contributed to the death.
4. Toxicology Tests: Samples of blood, urine, and other bodily fluids are taken to perform toxicology tests to determine the presence of drugs, alcohol, or other substances that may have contributed to the child's death.
5. Histological Examination: Samples of tissue are taken

and analyzed under a microscope to detect abnormalities that may have contributed to the death.

6. Final Report: After the autopsy is completed, a final report is generated that includes the cause and manner of death. This report is provided to the family, and it may also be used in legal proceedings, research, or educational purposes.

Autopsies can be a valuable tool in providing closure for families and preventing future deaths. The information gathered from an autopsy can be used to develop preventative measures, educate the medical community, and improve patient care. It is essential that the autopsy process is handled with sensitivity, respect, and professionalism to ensure that families receive the answers and support they need during a difficult time.

CHAPTER 18

Physical Medicine and Rehabilitation

P ediatric Physical Medicine and Rehabilitation (PM&R) is a medical specialty that focuses on the diagnosis, treatment, and management of children with physical and functional disabilities resulting from congenital conditions, developmental disorders, injuries, or illnesses. The goal of pediatric PM&R is to improve the child's quality of life and functionality by addressing their physical, emotional, and social needs.

Common diagnoses that pediatric PM&R specialists treat include:

1. Cerebral Palsy: This is a group of motor disorders that affect muscle tone, movement, and coordination, resulting in difficulty with walking, sitting, and standing.
2. Spina Bifida: A congenital condition where the spinal cord does not develop properly, resulting in varying degrees of paralysis, bowel and bladder dysfunction, and other neurological complications.
3. Traumatic Brain Injury: This can occur as a result of an accident or sports injury and can cause long-term motor, cognitive, and behavioral impairments.
4. Neuromuscular Disorders: These include muscular dystrophy, spinal muscular atrophy, and myasthenia

gravis, which can cause muscle weakness, atrophy, and difficulty with movement.

5.   Sports Injuries: Pediatric PM&R specialists can help manage and rehabilitate a wide range of sports-related injuries, such as fractures, sprains, and concussions.

6.   Developmental Delays: These can result from a variety of factors, including genetic disorders, prematurity, and environmental factors, and can affect motor skills, speech, and cognitive development.

7.   Spinal Cord Injury: These can occur as a result of accidents or illnesses, and can cause partial or complete paralysis and other complications.

Pediatric PM&R specialists use a variety of techniques and treatments to help children improve their physical functioning, including physical therapy, occupational therapy, speech therapy, assistive devices, medications, and surgery. They work closely with other medical professionals, such as pediatricians, neurologists, and orthopedic surgeons, to provide comprehensive care and support for children with physical disabilities.

Cerebral Palsy

Cerebral palsy (CP) is a group of neurological disorders that affect movement and posture. CP is caused by damage to the brain that occurs before, during, or shortly after birth. The damage to the brain can lead to difficulties with muscle control, coordination, balance, and other motor functions. In this response, we will discuss pediatric cerebral palsy in detail, including its symptoms, causes, diagnosis, and treatment options.

Symptoms of Pediatric Cerebral Palsy: The symptoms of pediatric cerebral palsy can vary depending on the type and severity of the disorder. Some common symptoms of CP include:

1. Muscle stiffness or spasticity: Children with CP may experience muscle stiffness or spasticity, which can make it difficult to move their limbs or maintain good posture.
2. Weakness: Children with CP may also experience muscle weakness, which can make it difficult to perform certain tasks, such as holding a spoon or writing.
3. Coordination difficulties: Children with CP may have difficulties with coordination and balance, which can make it challenging to perform tasks that require precise movements.
4. Speech and language difficulties: Children with CP may also experience difficulties with speech and language, including slurred speech or difficulty with articulation.
5. Intellectual and developmental disabilities: Children with CP may be at increased risk for intellectual and developmental disabilities, which can impact their cognitive and social functioning.

Causes of Cerebral Palsy: The causes of pediatric cerebral palsy are complex and multifactorial. Some common causes of CP include:

1. Brain Damage: Cerebral palsy is caused by damage to the brain that occurs before, during, or shortly after birth. This damage can be caused by a range of factors, including genetic mutations, infections, or complications during delivery.
2. Premature Birth: Premature birth is a significant risk factor for cerebral palsy, as the brain may not have fully developed before the baby is born.
3. Lack of Oxygen: Lack of oxygen during birth can also

cause brain damage, leading to cerebral palsy.

Diagnosis of Cerebral Palsy: Pediatric cerebral palsy is typically diagnosed through a comprehensive medical evaluation, including a physical exam and neurological assessment. Doctors may also use imaging tests, such as MRI or CT scans, to evaluate brain structure and function.

Treatment of Cerebral Palsy: The treatment of pediatric cerebral palsy depends on the specific type and severity of the disorder. Treatment options may include:

1. Physical Therapy: Physical therapy is the most common treatment for cerebral palsy. A physical therapist will work with the child to improve their strength, flexibility, and motor function through exercises and techniques designed to improve movement and posture.
2. Occupational Therapy: Occupational therapy can also be helpful in managing cerebral palsy, as it focuses on improving the child's ability to perform daily activities and tasks.
3. Speech and Language Therapy: Speech and language therapy can help children with cerebral palsy improve their communication skills and overcome speech and language difficulties.
4. Assistive Devices: Assistive devices, such as braces, wheelchairs, or communication devices, may also be helpful in managing cerebral palsy and improving the child's quality of life.
5. Medications: In some cases, medications such as muscle relaxants or anti-spasticity drugs may be prescribed to manage symptoms of cerebral palsy.

Cerebral palsy is a group of neurological disorders that affect movement and posture. The symptoms and causes of cerebral palsy can vary, and the treatment options depend on the specific type and severity of the disorder. Early intervention is essential to ensure the best outcomes for children with cerebral palsy, and it is important to seek professional help if you suspect that your child may be experiencing symptoms of the disorder.

Spina Bifida

Spina bifida is a birth defect that affects the spine and spinal cord. It occurs when the neural tube, which forms the brain and spinal cord, fails to close properly during fetal development. This can result in a range of symptoms, from mild to severe. In this response, we will discuss pediatric spina bifida in detail, including its types, causes, diagnosis, and treatment options.

Types of Spina Bifida: There are three main types of spina bifida:

1. Spina bifida occulta: This is the mildest form of spina bifida and occurs when one or more vertebrae do not close properly. The spinal cord is usually unaffected, and most people with spina bifida occulta do not experience any symptoms.

2. Meningocele: This form of spina bifida occurs when the meninges, the protective covering of the spinal cord, protrude through a gap in the vertebrae. This can result in a fluid-filled sac or bulge on the baby's back.

3. Myelomeningocele: This is the most severe form of spina bifida and occurs when the spinal cord and its protective covering protrude through a gap in the vertebrae. This can result in a fluid-filled sac or bulge on the baby's back, and the child may experience paralysis or other neurological problems.

Causes of Spina Bifida: The exact causes of spina bifida are not fully understood, but there are several risk factors that increase the likelihood of the condition occurring. Some common risk factors for spina bifida include:

1. Genetic factors: Spina bifida can run in families, and there may be a genetic component to the condition.
2. Folate deficiency: A lack of folic acid during pregnancy has been linked to an increased risk of spina bifida.
3. Certain medications: Some medications, such as anti-seizure medications, have been linked to an increased risk of spina bifida.
4. Environmental factors:Exposure to certain chemicals or toxins during pregnancy may increase the risk of spina bifida.

Diagnosis of Spina Bifida: Pediatric spina bifida is typically diagnosed through a combination of prenatal screening tests and diagnostic tests after birth. Prenatal screening tests may include blood tests or ultrasound imaging, which can detect abnormalities in the fetus. Diagnostic tests after birth may include an MRI or CT scan, which can evaluate the extent of the spinal cord defect.

Treatment of Spina Bifida: The treatment of pediatric spina bifida depends on the type and severity of the condition. Some treatment options may include:

1. Surgery: Surgery may be necessary to close the opening in the vertebrae and repair any damage to the spinal cord. This is usually done within the first few days of life for babies with myelomeningocele.
2. Shunts: Children with hydrocephalus, a condition in which there is excess fluid in the brain, may need a shunt to drain the fluid and reduce pressure on the brain.
3. Physical Therapy: Physical therapy can help children with spina bifida improve their strength and mobility, and

learn to manage any physical disabilities.

4.   Occupational Therapy: Occupational therapy can help children with spina bifida learn to perform daily activities and tasks independently.

5.   Assistive Devices: Assistive devices, such as braces, crutches, or wheelchairs, may be necessary to help children with spina bifida manage their physical disabilities and improve their quality of life.

Spina bifida is a birth defect that affects the spine and spinal cord. The type and severity of the condition can vary, and the treatment options

Traumatic Brain Injury

Traumatic brain injury (TBI) refers to damage to the brain caused by a physical blow, jolt, or bump to the head that disrupts normal brain function. This can result in a range of symptoms and long-term effects, from mild to severe. In this response, we will discuss pediatric traumatic brain injury in detail, including its causes, symptoms, diagnosis, and treatment options.

Causes of Traumatic Brain Injury: traumatic brain injury can be caused by a variety of events, including:

1.   Falls: Falls are the most common cause of pediatric traumatic brain injury, particularly in young children.
2.   Motor Vehicle Accidents: Car accidents are a common cause of pediatric traumatic brain injury, particularly in older children and adolescents.
3.   Sports Injuries: Contact sports, such as football, hockey, and soccer, can result in pediatric traumatic brain injury.
4.   Physical Abuse:

Shaken baby syndrome, which occurs when a baby is shaken violently, can cause traumatic brain injury.

Symptoms of Traumatic Brain Injury: The symptoms of pediatric traumatic brain injury can vary depending on the severity of the injury, but may include:

1. Headache: A headache is a common symptom of pediatric traumatic brain injury.
2. Nausea and Vomiting: Nausea and vomiting may occur after a pediatric traumatic brain injury.
3. Seizures: Seizures can occur in children with traumatic brain injury, particularly if the injury is severe.
4. Loss of Consciousness: Loss of consciousness may occur immediately after the injury, or several hours or days later.
5. Mood Changes: Children with traumatic brain injury may experience mood changes, such as irritability, sadness, or anxiety.

Diagnosis of Traumatic Brain Injury: Pediatric traumatic brain injury is typically diagnosed through a combination of physical examination and diagnostic tests, such as a CT scan or MRI. These tests can help to evaluate the extent of the injury and determine the best course of treatment.

Treatment of Traumatic Brain Injury: The treatment of pediatric traumatic brain injury depends on the severity of the injury and the specific symptoms that the child is experiencing. Some treatment options may include:

1. Observation: Mild cases of pediatric traumatic brain injury may require only observation and monitoring of symptoms.
2. Medications: Medications may be used to manage symptoms such as headaches, seizures, or mood changes.
3. Surgery: Surgery may be necessary to relieve pressure on the brain, remove blood clots, or repair damage to the skull.
4. Rehabilitation: Rehabilitation, including physical

therapy, occupational therapy, and speech therapy, may be necessary to help children recover from traumatic brain injury and regain their functional abilities.

5. Supportive Care: Supportive care, such as providing a quiet environment, managing pain, and providing emotional support, can also be important in the management of pediatric traumatic brain injury.

Traumatic brain injury is a serious condition that can result in a range of symptoms and long-term effects. It can be caused by a variety of events, including falls, sports injuries, and physical abuse. The treatment of pediatric traumatic brain injury depends on the severity of the injury and the specific symptoms that the child is experiencing, but may include observation, medications, surgery, rehabilitation, and supportive care. Early recognition and appropriate treatment are critical to the long-term outcome for children with traumatic brain injury.

Neuromuscular Disorders

Neuromuscular disorders are a group of conditions that affect the muscles and nerves that control movement in children. These disorders can be caused by genetic or acquired factors and can lead to a wide range of symptoms and functional impairments. In this response, we will discuss pediatric neuromuscular disorders in detail, including their causes, symptoms, diagnosis, and treatment options.

Causes of Neuromuscular Disorders: Pediatric neuromuscular disorders can be caused by genetic or acquired factors. Some common genetic causes of neuromuscular disorders include:

1. Muscular Dystrophy: This is a group of genetic disorders that cause progressive muscle weakness and wasting.
2. Spinal Muscular Atrophy: This is a genetic disorder that causes progressive weakness and wasting of the muscles.

3. Charcot-Marie-Tooth Disease: This is a genetic disorder that affects the peripheral nerves, leading to muscle weakness and wasting.

Acquired causes of pediatric neuromuscular disorders include:

1. Guillain-Barre Syndrome: This is an autoimmune disorder that affects the peripheral nerves, leading to muscle weakness and paralysis.
2. Polio: This is a viral infection that can cause muscle weakness and paralysis.

Symptoms of Neuromuscular Disorders: The symptoms of pediatric neuromuscular disorders can vary depending on the specific disorder and the severity of the condition. Some common symptoms of neuromuscular disorders in children include:

1. Muscle Weakness: This is the most common symptom of neuromuscular disorders in children and can affect any part of the body.
2. Muscle Wasting: Muscle wasting occurs when muscle tissue is lost due to lack of use or damage to the nerves that control the muscles.
3. Difficulty Walking: Children with neuromuscular disorders may have difficulty walking or may require the use of assistive devices such as braces or wheelchairs.
4. Fatigue: Children with neuromuscular disorders may tire easily and have reduced stamina.

Diagnosis of Neuromuscular Disorders: The diagnosis of pediatric neuromuscular disorders typically involves a combination of physical examination, medical history, and diagnostic tests. Some common diagnostic tests used to diagnose neuromuscular disorders in children include:

1. Electromyography (EMG): This test measures the electrical activity of muscles and can help to diagnose

muscle and nerve disorders.
2.   Nerve Conduction Studies: This test measures how well the nerves that control muscles are functioning.
3.   Genetic Testing: This test can help to identify genetic causes of neuromuscular disorders.

Treatment of Neuromuscular Disorders: The treatment of pediatric neuromuscular disorders depends on the specific disorder and the severity of the condition. Some common treatment options for neuromuscular disorders in children include:

1.   Medications: Medications can be used to manage symptoms such as muscle weakness, pain, and fatigue.
2.   Physical Therapy: Physical therapy can help to improve muscle strength and flexibility and promote functional independence.
3.   Braces and Assistive Devices: Braces and other assistive devices such as wheelchairs and walkers can help to improve mobility and functional independence.
4.   Surgery: Surgery may be necessary to correct skeletal abnormalities or to release tight muscles and tendons.
5.   Supportive Care: Supportive care, including respiratory support, nutritional support, and emotional support, can be important in the management of pediatric neuromuscular disorders.

Neuromuscular disorders are a group of conditions that affect the muscles and nerves that control movement in children. They can be caused by genetic or acquired factors and can lead to a wide range of symptoms and functional impairments. The diagnosis and treatment of pediatric neuromuscular disorders depend on the specific disorder and the severity

Sports Injuries

Pediatric sports injuries are injuries that occur during sports or physical activity in children and adolescents. These injuries can range from mild to severe and can affect different parts of the body. In this response, we will discuss pediatric sports injuries in detail, including their causes, symptoms, prevention, and treatment options.

Causes of Sports Injuries:Pediatric sports injuries can be caused by a variety of factors, including:

1.   Overuse: Overuse injuries occur when a particular body part is used repeatedly without enough time to rest and recover.
2.   Trauma: Traumatic injuries occur when there is a sudden force or impact on a body part, such as a fall, collision, or contact with an object.
3.   Improper Technique: Using improper technique during sports or physical activity can lead to injuries.
4.   Lack of Conditioning: Lack of conditioning can lead to fatigue, which can increase the risk of injuries.

Common Sports Injuries: Some common pediatric sports injuries include:

1.   Sprains and Strains: Sprains occur when the ligaments that connect bones are stretched or torn, while strains occur when muscles or tendons are stretched or torn.
2.   Fractures: Fractures are breaks in bones and can range from mild to severe.
3.   Concussions: Concussions are a type of traumatic brain injury that can occur during sports or physical activity.
4.   Overuse Injuries: Overuse injuries can include conditions such as shin splints, stress fractures, and tendinitis.

Symptoms of Sports Injuries: The symptoms of pediatric sports injuries can vary depending on the type and severity of the injury. Some common symptoms of sports injuries in children include:

1.   Pain: Pain is the most common symptom of sports injuries in children.
2.   Swelling: Swelling can occur when there is inflammation in the affected area.
3.   Limited Range of Motion: Injuries can cause stiffness or limited range of motion in the affected area.
4.   Bruising: Bruising can occur when blood vessels are damaged due to an injury.

Prevention of Sports Injuries: Preventing pediatric sports injuries involves several strategies, including:

1.   Proper Technique: Using proper technique during sports or physical activity can help to prevent injuries.
2.   Warm-up and Cool-down: Warming up before physical activity and cooling down afterward can help to prevent injuries.
3.   Adequate Rest and Recovery: Taking time to rest and recover between activities can help to prevent overuse injuries.
4.   Proper Equipment: Wearing proper equipment, such as helmets, padding, and shoes, can help to prevent injuries.

Treatment of Sports Injuries: The treatment of pediatric sports injuries depends on the type and severity of the injury. Some common treatment options for pediatric sports injuries include:

1.   Rest: Resting the affected area is often the first step in treating sports injuries in children.
2.   Ice and Compression: Applying ice and compression to the affected area can help to reduce swelling and pain.
3.   Medications: Medications such as pain relievers and anti-inflammatories may be used to manage pain and inflammation.

4.   Physical Therapy: Physical therapy can help to improve range of motion, strength, and flexibility in the affected area.

5.   Surgery: Surgery may be necessary for severe injuries such as fractures or torn ligaments.

Sports injuries are common and can be caused by a variety of factors. The prevention and treatment of pediatric sports injuries involve several strategies, including using proper technique, warming up and cooling down, taking adequate rest and recovery, wearing proper equipment, and seeking prompt medical attention when necessary. By taking these steps, children can enjoy sports and physical activity safely and reduce their risk of injury.

Developmental Delays

Developmental delays refer to a significant delay or lag in a child's cognitive, motor, social, or emotional development compared to the typical development of other children of the same age. In this response, we will discuss pediatric developmental delays in detail, including their causes, symptoms, diagnosis, treatment, and prevention options.

Causes of Developmental Delays: Pediatric developmental delays can be caused by a variety of factors, including:

1.   Genetic factors: Some developmental delays may be caused by genetic factors such as Down syndrome, Fragile X syndrome, or other genetic disorders.

2.   Premature birth: Premature birth can increase the risk of developmental delays due to the immaturity of the baby's brain and body systems.

3.   Medical conditions: Some medical conditions such as hearing loss, vision impairment, or neurological disorders can lead to developmental delays.

4.   Environmental factors: Environmental factors such as malnutrition, neglect, or exposure to toxins can affect a child's development.

Symptoms of Developmental Delays: The symptoms of pediatric developmental delays can vary depending on the type and severity of the delay. Some common symptoms of developmental delays in children include:

1.   Delayed milestones: A child may not achieve developmental milestones such as sitting up, crawling, or walking at the expected age.
2.   Communication difficulties: A child may have difficulty with speech or language development.
3.   Behavioral issues: A child may display challenging behaviors such as aggression, impulsivity, or hyperactivity.
4.   Social difficulties: A child may have difficulty with social interactions, making friends, or understanding social cues.

Diagnosis of Developmental Delays: Diagnosing pediatric developmental delays typically involves a comprehensive evaluation of the child's developmental history, medical history, physical examination, and developmental assessments. Developmental assessments may include standardized tests to assess the child's cognitive, motor, speech, and social-emotional development.

Treatment of Developmental Delays: The treatment of pediatric developmental delays depends on the type and severity of the delay. Some common treatment options for developmental delays in children include:

1.   Early intervention services: Early intervention services such as speech therapy, occupational therapy, or physical therapy can help to improve developmental outcomes.
2.   Behavioral therapy: Behavioral therapy can help to

address challenging behaviors and improve social skills.
3. Medical treatment: Medical treatment such as medication or surgery may be necessary for certain medical conditions that contribute to developmental delays.
4. Assistive devices:Assistive devices such as hearing aids, glasses, or mobility aids can help to improve functioning.

Prevention of Developmental Delays:Preventing pediatric developmental delays involves several strategies, including:

1. Prenatal care: Getting adequate prenatal care can help to identify and manage risk factors for developmental delays.
2. Early identification: Identifying developmental delays early can help to facilitate early intervention services and improve outcomes.
3. Nutritious diet: Providing a nutritious diet can help to support optimal brain development.
4. Safe environment: Providing a safe and nurturing environment can help to reduce the risk of environmental factors contributing to developmental delays.

Developmental delays can have a significant impact on a child's development and functioning. The causes, symptoms, diagnosis, treatment, and prevention of pediatric developmental delays involve a multidisciplinary approach, including medical evaluation, developmental assessment, early intervention services, behavioral therapy, medical treatment, and assistive devices. By taking these steps, children with developmental delays can receive the support and interventions they need to achieve their full potential.

Spinal Cord Injury

Pediatric spinal cord injury refers to damage to the spinal cord in children under the age of 18. The spinal cord is a complex network of nerves that carries signals between the brain and the rest of the body. Damage to the spinal cord can result in temporary or permanent changes in a child's motor, sensory, or autonomic function. In this response, we will discuss pediatric spinal cord injury in detail, including its causes, symptoms, diagnosis, treatment, and prevention options.

Causes of Spinal Cord Injury: Pediatric spinal cord injury can be caused by a variety of factors, including:

1. Trauma: Trauma is the most common cause of spinal cord injury in children. Trauma can be caused by motor vehicle accidents, falls, sports injuries, or physical abuse.
2. Medical conditions: Some medical conditions such as cancer or infections can cause spinal cord injury in children.
3. Congenital disorders: Some congenital disorders such as spina bifida can cause spinal cord injury in children.

Symptoms of Spinal Cord Injury: The symptoms of pediatric spinal cord injury depend on the location and severity of the injury. Some common symptoms of spinal cord injury in children include:

1. Loss of sensation: A child may experience loss of sensation in their limbs or other areas of the body.
2. Loss of motor function: A child may experience paralysis or weakness in their limbs or other areas of the body.
3. Loss of bladder or bowel control: A child may experience loss of bladder or bowel control.
4. Breathing difficulties: A child may experience difficulty breathing due to the involvement of the respiratory muscles.

Diagnosis of Spinal Cord Injury: Diagnosing pediatric spinal cord injury typically involves a comprehensive evaluation of the child's medical history, physical examination, and imaging studies such as X-rays, MRI or CT scans. Additional tests may be performed to assess the child's neurological function, including sensory, motor, and autonomic function.

Treatment of Spinal Cord Injury: The treatment of pediatric spinal cord injury depends on the location and severity of the injury. Some common treatment options for spinal cord injury in children include:

1. Immobilization: Immobilization of the spine using braces, casts, or traction can help to stabilize the spine and prevent further injury.
2. Surgery: Surgery may be necessary to decompress the spinal cord, stabilize the spine, or repair any damage to the spinal cord.
3. Rehabilitation: Rehabilitation therapy such as physical therapy, occupational therapy, or speech therapy can help to improve the child's function and quality of life.
4. Medication: Pain medication or muscle relaxants may be prescribed to manage symptoms.

Prevention of Spinal Cord Injury: Preventing pediatric spinal cord injury involves several strategies, including:

1. Safe environment: Providing a safe environment for children can help to reduce the risk of falls, sports injuries, or physical abuse.
2. Proper use of car seats and seat belts: Proper use of car seats and seat belts can help to reduce the risk of spinal cord injury in motor vehicle accidents.
3. Sports safety: Using proper safety equipment and following sports safety guidelines can help to reduce the risk of spinal cord injury in sports.

Spinal cord injury can have a significant impact on a child's function and quality of life. The causes, symptoms, diagnosis, treatment, and prevention of pediatric spinal cord injury involve a multidisciplinary approach, including medical evaluation, imaging studies, immobilization, surgery, rehabilitation, medication, and prevention strategies. By taking these steps, children with spinal cord injury can receive the support and interventions they need to achieve their full potential.

CHAPTER 19

Emergency Medicine

Pediatric emergency medicine is a medical specialty that focuses on the diagnosis, treatment, and management of acutely ill or injured children. This field of medicine requires specialized training and knowledge to handle the unique needs of pediatric patients. Pediatric emergency medicine physicians work in emergency departments, urgent care clinics, and other healthcare settings that provide urgent and emergent care for children.

Common diagnoses treated in pediatric emergency medicine include:

1.   Respiratory Distress: This can be caused by a variety of factors, including asthma, bronchitis, pneumonia, and other respiratory infections.
2.   Seizures: These can occur due to a variety of reasons, including epilepsy, febrile seizures, and head injuries.
3.   Dehydration: This can occur due to vomiting, diarrhea, or inadequate fluid intake and can lead to electrolyte imbalances, hypovolemia, and shock.
4.   Traumatic Injuries: These can include fractures, lacerations, burns, and head injuries, which can result from accidents, falls, or sports-related injuries.
5.   Gastrointestinal Disorders: These can include appendicitis, gastroenteritis, and inflammatory bowel

disease.

6.   Allergic Reactions: These can range from mild allergic reactions to life-threatening anaphylaxis and can be triggered by food, medications, or insect bites.

7.   Poisonings: These can be caused by a variety of substances, including medications, household cleaners, and pesticides.

Pediatric emergency medicine physicians use a variety of diagnostic and treatment techniques to care for acutely ill or injured children. These can include imaging tests, laboratory tests, medications, and procedures such as intubation, CPR, and suturing. They work closely with other healthcare professionals, such as nurses, respiratory therapists, and pediatricians, to provide comprehensive care and support for children in emergency situations.

Respiratory Distress

Respiratory distress is a common reason for children to present to the emergency room (ER). Respiratory distress can be caused by a variety of conditions, including asthma, bronchiolitis, pneumonia, and croup. In this response, I will discuss some of the common causes of pediatric respiratory distress seen in the ER, their clinical presentation, and management.

1.   Asthma: Asthma is a chronic lung condition characterized by airway inflammation and hyperresponsiveness. Children with asthma may present with symptoms such as wheezing, coughing, shortness of breath, and chest tightness. Treatment in the ER may involve administering bronchodilators, corticosteroids, and oxygen therapy.

2.   Bronchiolitis: Bronchiolitis is a viral infection that affects the small airways in the lungs. Children with bronchiolitis may present with symptoms such as

coughing, wheezing, and difficulty breathing. Treatment in the ER may involve administering oxygen therapy, suctioning the airways to remove secretions, and providing supportive care.

3.   Pneumonia: Pneumonia is a bacterial or viral infection that affects the lungs. Children with pneumonia may present with symptoms such as coughing, fever, chest pain, and difficulty breathing. Treatment in the ER may involve administering antibiotics, oxygen therapy, and providing supportive care.

4.   Croup: Croup is a viral infection that affects the larynx and trachea. Children with croup may present with symptoms such as a barking cough, hoarseness, and difficulty breathing. Treatment in the ER may involve administering nebulized epinephrine, corticosteroids, and oxygen therapy.

5.   Foreign body aspiration: Foreign body aspiration occurs when a child inhales an object into their airway. Children with foreign body aspiration may present with symptoms such as choking, coughing, and difficulty breathing. Treatment in the ER may involve removing the object from the airway through techniques such as suctioning or bronchoscopy.

Pediatric respiratory distress is a common reason for children to present to the emergency room. Treatment in the ER depends on the underlying cause of the respiratory distress and may involve administering medications such as bronchodilators or antibiotics, providing oxygen therapy, and providing supportive care. Early recognition and management of pediatric respiratory distress can help prevent serious complications and improve outcomes.

Seizures

Seizures are a common reason for children to present to the

emergency room (ER). Seizures can be caused by a variety of conditions, including epilepsy, fever, head injury, and infections. In this response, I will discuss some of the common causes of pediatric seizures seen in the ER, their clinical presentation, and management.

1. Febrile seizures: Febrile seizures are seizures that occur in children with a fever. They typically occur in children between the ages of 6 months and 5 years. Febrile seizures may be generalized or focal and can last for a few seconds to several minutes. Treatment in the ER may involve giving medications such as acetaminophen or ibuprofen to reduce the fever and administering benzodiazepines to stop the seizure.

2. Epileptic seizures: Epileptic seizures are seizures that occur due to abnormal electrical activity in the brain. Children with epilepsy may experience a variety of seizure types, including generalized tonic-clonic seizures, absence seizures, and focal seizures. Treatment in the ER may involve giving antiepileptic medications, such as benzodiazepines or phenytoin, to stop the seizure.

3. Head injury seizures: Seizures can occur after a head injury, especially if there is bleeding or swelling in the brain. Treatment in the ER may involve stabilizing the child's airway and administering antiepileptic medications if necessary.

4. Infection-related seizures: Seizures can occur in children with infections such as meningitis or encephalitis. Treatment in the ER may involve administering antibiotics or antiviral medications to treat the infection and giving antiepileptic medications to stop the seizure.

5. Metabolic disorders: Some metabolic disorders, such as hypoglycemia or electrolyte imbalances, can cause seizures. Treatment in the ER may involve correcting the underlying metabolic abnormality and administering antiepileptic medications to stop the seizure.

Seizures are a common reason for children to present to the emergency room. Treatment in the ER depends on the underlying cause of the seizure and may involve giving medications such as benzodiazepines or antiepileptic medications, stabilizing the child's airway, and providing supportive care. Early recognition and management of pediatric seizures can help prevent serious complications and improve outcomes.

Dehydration

Dehydration is a common reason for children to present to the emergency room (ER). Dehydration occurs when a child loses more fluids than they take in, and can be caused by conditions such as vomiting, diarrhea, fever, or inadequate fluid intake. In this response, I will discuss the clinical presentation and management of pediatric dehydration in the ER.

Clinical presentation: Children with dehydration may present with symptoms such as dry mouth, sunken eyes, decreased urine output, lethargy, and irritability. In severe cases, children may have a rapid heart rate, low blood pressure, and signs of shock.

Management: The goal of management in the ER is to rehydrate the child and correct any underlying causes of dehydration. Treatment may involve:

1. Oral rehydration therapy: If the child is able to tolerate oral fluids, oral rehydration therapy (ORT) may be initiated. ORT involves giving the child small amounts of fluids containing electrolytes, such as Pedialyte, every few minutes until they are able to tolerate larger amounts.
2. Intravenous fluids: If the child is unable to tolerate oral fluids or has severe dehydration, they may require intravenous (IV) fluids. The type and amount of fluids

given will depend on the child's weight and severity of dehydration.

3.   Treatment of underlying causes: If the dehydration is caused by an underlying condition such as vomiting or diarrhea, the underlying cause will be treated.

4.   Monitoring: Children with dehydration will need close monitoring in the ER. Vital signs, urine output, and electrolyte levels will be closely monitored to ensure that the child is adequately rehydrated.

Prevention: Prevention of dehydration is key in avoiding the need for emergency treatment. Encouraging children to drink fluids regularly, especially during periods of illness, can help prevent dehydration. In cases of diarrhea or vomiting, providing electrolyte-rich fluids such as Pedialyte can help prevent dehydration.

Dehydration is a common reason for children to present to the emergency room. Management in the ER involves rehydration and correction of any underlying causes of dehydration. Prevention of dehydration is important in avoiding the need for emergency treatment.

Traumatic Injuries

Pediatric traumatic injuries are a common reason for children to present to the emergency room (ER). Traumatic injuries in children can be caused by a variety of factors, including falls, sports-related injuries, motor vehicle accidents, and physical abuse. In this response, I will discuss some of the common types of pediatric traumatic injuries seen in the ER, their clinical presentation, and management.

1.   Head injuries: Head injuries are a common type of pediatric injury that can range from mild concussions to severe traumatic brain injuries. Symptoms of head injuries may include headache, vomiting, confusion,

dizziness, or loss of consciousness. Treatment in the ER may involve imaging studies such as a CT scan or MRI to assess the severity of the injury and close monitoring of the child's vital signs.

2.   Fractures: Fractures are another common type of pediatric injury, especially in the arms and legs. Clinical presentation may include pain, swelling, and deformity. Treatment in the ER may involve splinting or casting the affected area to immobilize the fracture and manage pain.

3.   Abdominal injuries: Abdominal injuries can occur due to motor vehicle accidents or physical abuse. Clinical presentation may include abdominal pain, nausea, vomiting, and signs of shock. Treatment in the ER may involve imaging studies such as a CT scan to assess the severity of the injury and surgical intervention if necessary.

4.   Burns: Burns can occur due to exposure to hot liquids, flames, or chemicals. Clinical presentation may include redness, blistering, and pain. Treatment in the ER may involve cleaning the affected area, applying dressings, and administering pain management.

5.   Soft tissue injuries: Soft tissue injuries, such as cuts and bruises, can occur due to falls or sports-related injuries. Treatment in the ER may involve cleaning the affected area, applying dressings, and administering pain management.

Traumatic injuries are a common reason for children to present to the emergency room. Treatment in the ER depends on the type and severity of the injury and may involve imaging studies, surgical intervention, and pain management. Early recognition and management of pediatric traumatic injuries can help prevent serious complications and improve outcomes.

Gastrointestinal Disorders

Gastrointestinal disorders are a common reason for children to present to the emergency room (ER). These disorders can range from minor conditions, such as gastroenteritis, to more serious and potentially life-threatening conditions, such as intussusception or necrotizing enterocolitis. In this response, I will discuss some of the common pediatric gastrointestinal disorders that present to the ER, their clinical presentation, and management.

1.   Gastroenteritis: Gastroenteritis is an inflammation of the gastrointestinal tract, usually caused by a viral or bacterial infection. Children with gastroenteritis typically present with vomiting, diarrhea, and abdominal pain. Treatment in the ER usually consists of rehydration with intravenous fluids, antiemetics to control vomiting, and analgesics to control abdominal pain.

2.   Appendicitis: Appendicitis is an inflammation of the appendix, a small organ attached to the large intestine. Children with appendicitis typically present with abdominal pain, nausea, and vomiting. In some cases, the pain may begin around the belly button and then move to the right lower abdomen. Treatment for appendicitis usually involves surgical removal of the appendix.

3.   Intussusception: Intussusception occurs when one part of the intestine slides into an adjacent part, causing a blockage. Children with intussusception typically present with severe abdominal pain, vomiting, and bloody stools. Treatment usually involves an air enema or surgery.

4.   Malrotation: Malrotation occurs when the intestines do not properly rotate and position themselves during fetal development. Children with malrotation may present with vomiting, abdominal distention, and bloody stools. Treatment usually involves surgery to correct the malrotation.

5.   Necrotizing enterocolitis (NEC): NEC is a serious

intestinal condition that primarily affects premature infants. Children with NEC may present with vomiting, bloody stools, abdominal distention, and lethargy. Treatment usually involves hospitalization, intravenous antibiotics, and surgical intervention in severe cases.

Gastrointestinal disorders are a common reason for children to present to the ER. The clinical presentation and management of these disorders can vary widely, depending on the specific condition. Timely and appropriate management in the ER is crucial to prevent complications and improve outcomes.

Allergic Reactions

Allergic reactions can range from mild symptoms such as hives and itching to severe and life-threatening conditions such as anaphylaxis. When a child presents to the emergency room (ER) with an allergic reaction, it is essential to determine the severity of the reaction and provide appropriate management. In this response, I will discuss the most common pediatric allergic reactions treated in the ER and their management.

1. Anaphylaxis: Anaphylaxis is a severe and potentially life-threatening allergic reaction that affects multiple organ systems. Children with anaphylaxis may present with symptoms such as swelling of the face, lips, and tongue, difficulty breathing, vomiting, and loss of consciousness. The first-line treatment for anaphylaxis is epinephrine, which is given as an injection. Other treatments may include intravenous fluids, antihistamines, and corticosteroids.

2. Asthma exacerbations: Asthma exacerbations are a common allergic reaction that can cause severe breathing difficulties in children. Children with asthma exacerbations may present with wheezing, shortness

of breath, coughing, and chest tightness. Treatment for asthma exacerbations in the ER may include bronchodilators, corticosteroids, and oxygen therapy.

3.   Urticaria (hives): Urticaria is a skin rash characterized by raised, itchy, and red bumps. Children with urticaria may present with mild to severe symptoms, depending on the severity of the reaction. Treatment for urticaria may include antihistamines and corticosteroids.

4.   Angioedema: Angioedema is a swelling of the deeper layers of the skin and tissues, typically around the face and throat. Children with angioedema may present with difficulty breathing, speaking, or swallowing. Treatment for angioedema may include epinephrine, antihistamines, and corticosteroids.

5.   Food allergies: Food allergies can cause a wide range of symptoms, from mild to severe. Children with food allergies may present with symptoms such as hives, itching, nausea, vomiting, and abdominal pain. In severe cases, food allergies can cause anaphylaxis. Treatment for food allergies in the ER may include antihistamines, corticosteroids, and epinephrine.

Allergic reactions can be severe and life-threatening. In the ER, it is crucial to determine the severity of the reaction and provide appropriate management. Treatment may include medications such as antihistamines, corticosteroids, and epinephrine, as well as oxygen therapy and intravenous fluids. Timely and appropriate management can improve outcomes and prevent complications.

Poisonings

Pediatric poisonings are a common reason for children to

present to the emergency room (ER). Poisonings can occur from a variety of sources, including medications, household products, and plants. In this response, I will discuss some of the common pediatric poisonings seen in the ER, their clinical presentation, and management.

1. Medication poisonings: Medication poisonings can occur when children accidentally ingest or overdose on medications, including prescription and over-the-counter medications. Symptoms can vary depending on the type and amount of medication ingested but can include nausea, vomiting, dizziness, confusion, and difficulty breathing. Treatment in the ER may involve giving activated charcoal to absorb the medication, administering antidotes, and providing supportive care.

2. Household product poisonings: Household product poisonings can occur when children accidentally ingest or inhale products such as cleaning products, pesticides, and cosmetics. Symptoms can include nausea, vomiting, difficulty breathing, and seizures. Treatment in the ER may involve administering activated charcoal, providing oxygen, and giving intravenous fluids.

3. Carbon monoxide poisonings: Carbon monoxide is an odorless and colorless gas that can be deadly if inhaled in high concentrations. Children with carbon monoxide poisoning may present with symptoms such as headache, dizziness, nausea, and confusion. Treatment in the ER may involve giving oxygen and providing supportive care.

4. Plant poisonings: Plant poisonings can occur when children ingest or touch toxic plants such as poison ivy, poison oak, or poison sumac. Symptoms can include skin irritation, rash, vomiting, and diarrhea. Treatment in the ER may involve giving antihistamines, administering topical creams, and providing supportive care.

5. Lead poisonings: Lead poisoning can occur when children ingest or inhale lead from sources such as

old paint, contaminated soil, or toys. Symptoms can include developmental delays, learning difficulties, and abdominal pain. Treatment in the ER may involve administering chelation therapy to remove the lead from the child's body.

Poisonings can be serious and require immediate medical attention. In the ER, treatment may involve giving activated charcoal, providing oxygen, administering antidotes, and providing supportive care. Early recognition and management of pediatric poisonings can help prevent serious complications and improve outcomes.

CHAPTER 20

Neonatology

Neonatology is a subspecialty of pediatrics that focuses on the care of newborn infants, particularly those who are premature, critically ill, or have medical or surgical conditions that require specialized care. Neonatologists are pediatricians who have received additional training in the care of newborn infants and provide care in neonatal intensive care units (NICUs) and other specialized units.

Common diagnoses treated in neonatology include:

1. Prematurity: Infants born before 37 weeks of gestation may require specialized care to help them grow and develop. They may require respiratory support, nutritional support, and close monitoring for complications such as infection or brain injury.

2. Respiratory Distress Syndrome (RDS): This condition is caused by a lack of surfactant in the lungs, which makes it difficult for the baby to breathe. Infants with RDS may require oxygen therapy, mechanical ventilation, and medications to help with lung function.

3. Neonatal Jaundice: This is a common condition in newborns that occurs when there is an excess of bilirubin in the blood. Infants with jaundice may require phototherapy or exchange transfusions to lower the

bilirubin levels.

4.　　Infections: Newborns are particularly vulnerable to infections due to their immature immune systems. Common infections treated in neonatology include sepsis, meningitis, and pneumonia.

5.　　Congenital Heart Disease: Some infants are born with heart defects that require surgical or medical intervention to correct. Neonatologists work closely with pediatric cardiologists and cardiac surgeons to provide specialized care for infants with heart disease.

6.　　Neonatal Abstinence Syndrome (NAS): Infants born to mothers who used opioids during pregnancy may experience withdrawal symptoms after birth. Neonatologists can provide supportive care and medications to help manage these symptoms.

7.　　Birth Injuries: Some infants may experience injuries during delivery, such as brain injuries, nerve damage, or fractures. Neonatologists can provide specialized care for infants with birth injuries to help them recover and prevent long-term complications.

Neonatologists use a variety of diagnostic and treatment techniques to care for newborn infants, including advanced imaging tests, laboratory tests, and procedures such as intubation, ventilation, and surgery. They work closely with other healthcare professionals, such as nurses, respiratory therapists, and pediatric surgeons, to provide comprehensive care and support for newborn infants who require specialized care.

Prematurity

Prematurity is a term used to describe a newborn baby who is born before the completion of the 37th week of gestation. Premature birth is a significant public health concern worldwide and is associated with increased morbidity and mortality rates, particularly among very premature infants.

There are many causes of premature birth, including maternal factors such as infections, chronic diseases, and lifestyle factors such as smoking and drug use. Fetal factors such as multiple gestation and congenital anomalies may also contribute to premature birth.

Premature infants are at risk of a wide range of medical complications due to their underdeveloped organs and systems. Some of the most common complications associated with prematurity include:

1. Respiratory distress syndrome (RDS): This is a condition where the baby's lungs are not fully developed and cannot produce enough surfactant, a substance that helps to keep the lungs inflated. RDS can cause breathing difficulties and requires intensive medical support, including mechanical ventilation and oxygen therapy.

2. Apnea of prematurity: This is a condition where the baby stops breathing for a period of time. It is common in premature infants and may require monitoring and treatment with medication or respiratory support.

3. Intraventricular hemorrhage (IVH): This is bleeding in the brain that can occur in premature infants due to the fragility of their blood vessels. Severe cases of IVH can cause long-term neurological deficits and disabilities.

4. Retinopathy of prematurity (ROP): This is a disorder that affects the development of the blood vessels in the retina of premature infants. Severe cases can lead to blindness.

5. Necrotizing enterocolitis (NEC): This is a serious condition where the lining of the intestines becomes damaged and can lead to life-threatening complications such as infection and perforation.

6. Sepsis: Premature infants are at increased risk of infections due to their immature immune systems and prolonged hospital stays.

The management of prematurity requires a multidisciplinary approach involving neonatologists, pediatricians, nurses, respiratory therapists, and other healthcare providers. Treatment depends on the severity of the complications and may include respiratory support, nutritional support, and medication for various conditions.

In addition to medical treatment, premature infants require careful monitoring and support during their development. They may require specialized interventions such as physical therapy, occupational therapy, and speech therapy to address developmental delays and other complications.

Prematurity is a significant public health concern that can result in a wide range of medical complications for newborns. Effective management requires a multidisciplinary approach and ongoing support to address the unique needs of premature infants and promote their healthy development.

Neonatal Respiratory Distress Syndrome

Neonatal Respiratory Distress Syndrome (NRDS) is a condition that occurs in premature babies when their lungs have not yet fully developed. It is also known as hyaline membrane disease (HMD). This condition occurs due to a lack of surfactant in the lungs.

Surfactant is a substance that lines the inside of the lungs and helps them to stay open by reducing the surface tension. It is produced by the type II pneumocytes in the lungs and helps to prevent the collapse of the small air sacs (alveoli) in the lungs during exhalation.

In premature infants, the lungs are not fully developed, and the production of surfactant may be insufficient. This leads to an increased surface tension in the alveoli, causing them to collapse, and making it difficult for the baby to breathe. This is known as NRDS.

The signs and symptoms of NRDS include rapid breathing, grunting, flaring of nostrils, and retractions (pulling in of the chest muscles). The baby may also have low oxygen levels (hypoxemia) and a bluish tint to their skin (cyanosis).

The diagnosis of NRDS is made based on the baby's symptoms, physical examination, and laboratory tests such as blood gases and chest x-rays. Treatment involves providing oxygen and surfactant replacement therapy. Mechanical ventilation may also be needed in severe cases.

The prognosis for NRDS depends on the severity of the condition and the baby's overall health. With early diagnosis and treatment, the prognosis is generally good. However, if left untreated, NRDS can lead to complications such as lung damage, pneumonia, and respiratory failure.

NRDS is a condition that occurs in premature infants due to a lack of surfactant in the lungs, which can cause difficulty in breathing. Early diagnosis and treatment are essential for a good prognosis. The pathologist's role in the management of NRDS is to provide accurate diagnosis and interpretation of laboratory tests, including blood gases and chest x-rays.

Neonatal Jaundice

Neonatal jaundice is a common condition that occurs in newborns due to an accumulation of bilirubin in the blood. Bilirubin is a yellow pigment that is produced during the breakdown of red blood cells. In normal circumstances, bilirubin is eliminated from the body by the liver. However, in newborns, the liver may not be fully developed, leading to a buildup of bilirubin in the blood.

The symptoms of neonatal jaundice include yellowing of the skin and whites of the eyes, and the appearance of a yellow tint in the baby's urine and stools. In severe cases, the baby may be irritable, have difficulty feeding, and may develop a fever.

The diagnosis of neonatal jaundice is made by measuring the levels of bilirubin in the blood using a blood test. Treatment for neonatal jaundice depends on the severity of the condition. In mild cases, the condition may resolve on its own within a few days without any intervention. However, in more severe cases, treatment may involve phototherapy, which involves exposing the baby's skin to a special type of light that helps to break down bilirubin. In some cases, exchange transfusion may be required, where a small amount of the baby's blood is removed and replaced with fresh blood.

Neonatal jaundice is generally a benign condition, and most infants recover without any complications. However, in some cases, high levels of bilirubin can lead to complications such as kernicterus, a rare but serious condition that can cause brain damage and even death. It is important to monitor and manage neonatal jaundice appropriately to prevent complications.

Neonatal Infections

Neonatal infections are infections that occur in newborn infants within the first 28 days of life. These infections can be caused by a variety of pathogens, including bacteria, viruses, fungi, and parasites. Neonatal infections are a significant cause of morbidity and mortality in newborns, particularly those born prematurely or with a low birth weight.

Risk factors for neonatal infections include premature rupture of membranes, prolonged labor, maternal fever during labor, chorioamnionitis (inflammation of the placenta and membranes), and maternal colonization with Group B Streptococcus (GBS).

The symptoms of neonatal infections vary depending on the type of infection and the age of the infant. Common symptoms include fever, poor feeding, lethargy, respiratory distress, irritability, jaundice, and a bulging fontanelle (a soft spot on the baby's head). In some cases, the infection may be asymptomatic, making it difficult to diagnose.

Diagnosis of neonatal infections typically involves laboratory testing, including blood cultures, urine cultures, and cerebrospinal fluid (CSF) analysis. Treatment usually involves intravenous antibiotics, antivirals, or antifungals, depending on the type of infection. Supportive care, such as intravenous fluids and oxygen therapy, may also be necessary.

Prevention of neonatal infections is essential and involves several strategies, including good prenatal care, timely and appropriate treatment of maternal infections, and proper infection control practices in the neonatal intensive care unit (NICU).

Congenital Heart Disease

Congenital heart disease (CHD) is a group of heart defects that occur during fetal development and result in abnormalities of the heart's structure and function. It is the most common type of birth defect, affecting approximately 1 in 100 newborns. CHD can range from minor defects that do not require treatment to complex, life-threatening conditions that require immediate medical attention.

There are many different types of CHD, and the defects can occur in various parts of the heart. Some common types of CHD include:

1. Atrial septal defect (ASD): A hole in the wall (septum) that separates the two upper chambers (atria) of the heart.
2. Ventricular septal defect (VSD): A hole in the wall that separates the two lower chambers (ventricles) of the heart.
3. Patent ductus arteriosus (PDA): A blood vessel that connects the two major arteries leading from the heart does not close after birth.
4. Tetralogy of Fallot (TOF): A combination of four heart defects that affect blood flow through the heart and to the lungs.
5. Transposition of the great arteries (TGA): The two major arteries leading from the heart are reversed, so that the aorta originates from the right ventricle and the pulmonary artery originates from the left ventricle.

The causes of CHD are not fully understood, but they are thought to be a combination of genetic and environmental factors. Some genetic syndromes, such as Down syndrome and Turner syndrome, are associated with an increased risk of CHD. Other risk factors for CHD include maternal infections during pregnancy, certain medications taken during pregnancy, and maternal drug or alcohol use.

The symptoms of CHD vary depending on the type and severity of the defect. Some defects may not cause any symptoms, while others can cause cyanosis (a bluish tint to the skin), shortness of breath, fatigue, poor feeding, and failure to thrive.

Diagnosis of CHD typically involves a combination of physical examination, imaging tests (such as echocardiography), and cardiac catheterization. Treatment options for CHD depend on the type and severity of the defect, and may include medications, surgery, or catheter-based procedures.

In many cases, children with CHD require ongoing medical

care and monitoring throughout their lives. Some children may require additional surgeries or procedures as they grow and develop. With proper treatment and management, many children with CHD are able to lead healthy, active lives.

Neonatal Abstinence Syndrome

Neonatal abstinence syndrome (NAS) is a collection of symptoms that occurs in newborn infants who have been exposed to addictive drugs, such as opioids or benzodiazepines, while in the womb. The syndrome occurs due to the sudden withdrawal of these drugs from the infant's system once they are born.

Symptoms of NAS can vary widely depending on the type and amount of drug exposure. Common symptoms include tremors, irritability, excessive crying, poor feeding, vomiting, diarrhea, fever, sweating, and even seizures. Symptoms typically appear within 48 to 72 hours after birth, although they can sometimes appear up to two weeks after birth.

NAS is diagnosed by a combination of clinical assessment, drug screening of the mother and infant, and monitoring of the infant's symptoms. Treatment typically involves a combination of pharmacological and non-pharmacological interventions. Infants with severe symptoms may require medication to manage withdrawal symptoms, such as morphine or methadone. Non-pharmacological interventions, such as swaddling and breastfeeding, can also help soothe the infant and promote their overall health and development.

Long-term outcomes of NAS are variable and can depend on the severity and duration of drug exposure, as well as the quality of care received by the infant after birth. Some infants may experience developmental delays or behavioral problems, while others may have no long-term effects.

Prevention of NAS involves addressing the underlying cause of drug exposure in the mother, such as through addiction treatment and prenatal care. Early identification and management of NAS can also improve outcomes for affected infants. Close collaboration between obstetricians, neonatologists, pediatricians, and addiction specialists is essential to ensure the best possible care for both mother and infant.

Birth Injuries

Birth injuries are defined as any physical damage that occurs to an infant during the birth process. These injuries can range from mild to severe, and may have both short-term and long-term effects on the infant's health and well-being.

There are several different types of birth injuries that can occur, including:

1. Head injuries: These can include skull fractures, brain hemorrhages, and other injuries that occur as a result of trauma to the head during delivery.
2. Brachial plexus injuries: These injuries occur when the nerves that control movement in the arms and hands are damaged during delivery.
3. Shoulder dystocia: This occurs when the baby's shoulder gets stuck behind the mother's pubic bone during delivery, which can cause nerve damage, fractures, and other injuries.
4. Fractures: These can occur to any bone in the baby's body during delivery, but most commonly occur to the clavicle (collarbone).
5. Cerebral palsy: This is a neurological disorder that can result from brain damage that occurs during delivery. It can cause problems with movement, posture, and coordination.

The causes of birth injuries can vary widely, but some of the most common include:

1. Prolonged labor: When labor lasts for an extended period of time, it can put both the mother and baby at risk for injury.
2. Difficult delivery: If the baby is too large or in an awkward position, it can make delivery more difficult and increase the risk of injury.
3. Use of forceps or vacuum extraction: These tools can be helpful in delivering the baby, but they also carry an increased risk of injury.
4. Premature birth: Infants who are born prematurely are at increased risk for a wide range of health problems, including birth injuries.

CHAPTER 21

Psychiatry

Pediatric psychiatry is a specialized field of medicine that focuses on the diagnosis and treatment of mental health disorders in children and adolescents. Mental health disorders in children can have a significant impact on their development and quality of life. In this response, I will discuss some of the common mental health disorders diagnosed and treated in pediatric psychiatry.

1.   Attention Deficit Hyperactivity Disorder (ADHD): ADHD is a neurodevelopmental disorder characterized by symptoms of hyperactivity, impulsivity, and inattention. Treatment for ADHD may include medication and behavioral therapy.

2.   Anxiety Disorders: Anxiety disorders, such as generalized anxiety disorder, social anxiety disorder, and separation anxiety disorder, are common in children and can cause significant distress and impairment. Treatment may include cognitive-behavioral therapy, medication, and relaxation techniques.

3.   Depression: Depression is a common mental health disorder in children and adolescents characterized by feelings of sadness, hopelessness, and lack of interest in activities. Treatment may include medication, psychotherapy, and support from family and friends.

4.   Bipolar Disorder: Bipolar disorder is a mood disorder

characterized by episodes of mania and depression. Treatment may include mood stabilizing medication, therapy, and support from family and friends.

5.   Eating Disorders: Eating disorders, such as anorexia nervosa and bulimia nervosa, are serious mental health disorders that can have serious health consequences. Treatment may involve a combination of therapy, medication, and nutritional counseling.

6.   Autism Spectrum Disorder (ASD): ASD is a neurodevelopmental disorder characterized by impaired social interaction and communication skills. Treatment may include behavioral therapy, medication, and educational support.

7.   Post-Traumatic Stress Disorder (PTSD): PTSD is a mental health disorder that can develop in children who have experienced or witnessed a traumatic event. Treatment may involve psychotherapy, medication, and support from family and friends.

Pediatric psychiatry is an important field that focuses on the diagnosis and treatment of mental health disorders in children and adolescents. Common diagnoses treated in pediatric psychiatry include ADHD, anxiety disorders, depression, bipolar disorder, eating disorders, ASD, and PTSD. Early recognition and treatment of mental health disorders in children can have a significant impact on their development and quality of life.

Attention Deficit Hyperactivity Disorder

ADHD stands for Attention Deficit Hyperactivity Disorder, which is a neurodevelopmental disorder that affects children, adolescents, and adults. The condition is characterized by inattention, hyperactivity, and impulsivity, which can cause significant problems in daily life, such as academic and social difficulties. The symptoms of ADHD can vary widely from person to person, and the diagnosis is made by a medical professional, such as a pediatrician or psychiatrist.

Symptoms: The symptoms of ADHD can be divided into two categories: inattention and hyperactivity/impulsivity. A child may have predominantly one type of symptom, or both.

Inattention symptoms:

- Difficulty paying attention to details and making careless mistakes
- Difficulty staying focused on tasks or activities
- Trouble organizing tasks and activities
- Avoidance of tasks that require sustained mental effort
- Easily distracted by external stimuli
- Forgetfulness in daily activities
- Difficulty following through on instructions

Hyperactivity/Impulsivity symptoms:

- Fidgeting or squirming while seated
- Difficulty staying seated during activities when expected to
- Running or climbing excessively in inappropriate situations
- Difficulty engaging in leisure activities quietly
- Excessive talking or interrupting others
- Difficulty waiting for turns or delaying gratification
- Impulsive decision making and acting without considering consequences

Causes: The exact cause of ADHD is not fully understood, but there are several factors that are thought to contribute to the disorder. Some of these factors include:

- Genetics: ADHD is thought to have a strong genetic

component, with studies showing that the condition runs in families.

- Neurotransmitters: Neurotransmitters are chemicals in the brain that help regulate behavior. Research suggests that imbalances in certain neurotransmitters, such as dopamine and norepinephrine, may contribute to ADHD.
- Brain structure: Studies have found that people with ADHD have differences in the structure of certain parts of the brain, such as the prefrontal cortex, which is responsible for executive functioning and impulse control.
- Environmental factors: Factors such as prenatal exposure to alcohol or tobacco, premature birth, and low birth weight may also contribute to ADHD.

Treatment: There is no cure for ADHD, but treatment can help manage the symptoms and improve daily functioning. Treatment plans are typically individualized and may include a combination of medication, behavioral therapy, and lifestyle changes.

Medication: Stimulant medications, such as methylphenidate and amphetamines, are often prescribed to help manage the symptoms of ADHD. These medications work by increasing the levels of dopamine and norepinephrine in the brain, which can improve attention and impulse control. Non-stimulant medications, such as atomoxetine, may also be used.

Behavioral therapy: Behavioral therapy can help children with ADHD learn strategies to manage their symptoms and improve their functioning. Behavioral therapy may include parent training, social skills training, and individual therapy.

Lifestyle changes: Making changes to the child's daily routine and environment can also help manage symptoms of ADHD. Strategies such as establishing a consistent routine, creating a quiet study space, and minimizing distractions can all be helpful.

ADHD is a common neurodevelopmental disorder that affects children, adolescents, and adults. The symptoms of ADHD can be managed with a combination of medication, behavioral therapy, and lifestyle changes, which can improve daily functioning and overall quality of life.

Anxiety Disorders

Pediatric anxiety disorders are a group of mental health conditions that are characterized by excessive worry or fear that is out of proportion to the situation, and which interferes with a child's daily activities. Anxiety disorders can occur at any age, but they typically start in childhood or adolescence.

There are several different types of pediatric anxiety disorders, including:

1. Generalized anxiety disorder (GAD): This is characterized by excessive worry about a variety of everyday issues, such as school, family, friends, or health.
2. Separation anxiety disorder (SAD): This is characterized by excessive fear or worry about being away from parents or caregivers, and may cause a child to avoid school or other social situations.
3. Social anxiety disorder: This is characterized by intense fear or worry about social situations or being judged or scrutinized by others.
4. Panic disorder: This is characterized by sudden and unexpected attacks of intense fear or panic, which may be accompanied by physical symptoms such as racing heart, sweating, or shaking.
5. Specific phobias: These are intense fears of specific objects, situations, or activities, such as fear of heights,

animals, or flying.

Pediatric anxiety disorders are thought to be caused by a combination of genetic, environmental, and developmental factors. Children who have a family history of anxiety disorders, or who have experienced trauma or stressful life events, may be more likely to develop anxiety.

The symptoms of pediatric anxiety disorders can vary depending on the type of disorder, but may include:

- Excessive worry or fear that is out of proportion to the situation
- Physical symptoms such as sweating, trembling, or nausea
- Avoidance of certain situations or activities
- Difficulty sleeping or concentrating
- Irritability or restlessness
- Fatigue or lethargy
- Difficulty with school or social activities

Treatment for pediatric anxiety disorders typically involves a combination of therapy and medication. Cognitive-behavioral therapy (CBT) is a type of therapy that helps children learn to recognize and manage their anxious thoughts and behaviors. Medications such as selective serotonin reuptake inhibitors (SSRIs) may also be used to help manage symptoms.

Early intervention and treatment is important for children with anxiety disorders, as untreated anxiety can interfere with their academic, social, and emotional development. Parents and caregivers can help by providing a supportive and calm environment, encouraging open communication, and seeking professional help if necessary.

Depression

Depression is a mental health disorder that affects children and adolescents. It is a serious condition that can significantly impact a child's quality of life, social and academic functioning, and overall well being. Depression in children is different from sadness, which is a normal emotion experienced by everyone. Pediatric depression involves a persistent feeling of sadness, hopelessness, and lack of interest in activities that the child previously enjoyed.

The symptoms of depression can vary depending on the child's age and developmental stage. In younger children, symptoms may include irritability, clinginess, separation anxiety, and physical complaints such as stomach aches and headaches. Older children and adolescents may experience feelings of worthlessness, guilt, fatigue, difficulty concentrating, changes in appetite, and thoughts of death or suicide.

There are several risk factors associated with depression, including a family history of depression, chronic medical conditions, stressful life events, and exposure to trauma. The diagnosis of depression in children is typically made through a combination of clinical interviews, symptom questionnaires, and psychological testing.

Treatment for depression typically involves a combination of psychotherapy and medication. Psychotherapy is a form of talk therapy that helps children and adolescents understand their feelings and develop coping strategies. Cognitive-behavioral therapy (CBT) is a common form of psychotherapy used to treat depression in children. It involves teaching children how to identify and change negative thoughts and behaviors.

Antidepressant medications may also be prescribed for children and adolescents with depression. Selective serotonin reuptake inhibitors (SSRIs) are the most commonly used antidepressants in children. However, the use of antidepressants in children and adolescents is a topic of controversy and requires close monitoring by a qualified mental health professional.

In addition to psychotherapy and medication, lifestyle modifications can also be helpful in managing pediatric depression. Regular exercise, a healthy diet, and good sleep habits can all contribute to improved mental health.

Bipolar Disorder

Bipolar disorder is a psychiatric disorder that is characterized by unusual and intense shifts in mood, energy, and activity levels. It affects people of all ages, including children and adolescents. In the pediatric population, bipolar disorder is often referred to as pediatric bipolar disorder (PBD) or early-onset bipolar disorder (EOBD). The symptoms of PBD can be similar to those seen in adult bipolar disorder, but they can also be different.

Symptoms of PBD: The symptoms of PBD can be broadly classified into two categories: manic or hypomanic episodes and depressive episodes. The symptoms of mania or hypomania may include:

1. Extreme happiness or elation
2. Increased energy, restlessness, or agitation
3. Irritability or impatience
4. Decreased need for sleep
5. Rapid speech or racing thoughts
6. Grandiosity or inflated self-esteem
7. Poor judgment
8. Risk-taking behavior
9. Reckless behavior

The symptoms of depression may include:

1. Persistent sadness or hopelessness

2. Decreased interest in activities
3. Changes in appetite or sleep patterns
4. Fatigue or loss of energy
5. Feelings of worthlessness or guilt
6. Difficulty concentrating or making decisions
7. Suicidal thoughts or behavior

Diagnosis of PBD: The diagnosis of PBD is complex and requires a comprehensive evaluation by a qualified mental health professional. There are no laboratory tests or imaging studies that can diagnose bipolar disorder. A thorough medical and psychiatric history, as well as a detailed description of the patient's symptoms, is required. In some cases, family members or caregivers may also be interviewed to provide additional information.

Treatment of PBD: The treatment of PBD is multifaceted and may include a combination of pharmacotherapy and psychotherapy. The primary goal of treatment is to stabilize mood and reduce the frequency and severity of episodes. Mood stabilizers such as lithium, valproate, and carbamazepine are commonly used to treat PBD. Atypical antipsychotics such as risperidone, olanzapine, and aripiprazole may also be used. Psychotherapy, such as cognitive-behavioral therapy (CBT), family-focused therapy, and interpersonal and social rhythm therapy (IPSRT) may also be helpful in managing the symptoms of PBD.

Prognosis of PBD: The prognosis of PBD varies depending on the severity of symptoms, the age of onset, and the presence of comorbid conditions. Early diagnosis and treatment can help improve outcomes and reduce the risk of relapse. However, PBD can be a chronic and disabling condition that requires ongoing management and support.

Pediatric bipolar disorder is a complex psychiatric condition that requires a comprehensive evaluation and individualized treatment approach. Early diagnosis and treatment can help improve outcomes and reduce the risk of relapse.

Eating Disorders

Pediatric eating disorders refer to a group of psychiatric conditions characterized by disturbed eating habits and abnormal attitudes towards food and weight. These disorders commonly occur in children and adolescents, although they can affect individuals of any age group. Eating disorders can have serious consequences on a child's physical and mental health, and early diagnosis and treatment are crucial in preventing complications.

There are several types of eating disorders that commonly occur in pediatric patients, including:

1. Anorexia Nervosa: Anorexia is characterized by an extreme fear of weight gain, leading to self-starvation and a significantly low body weight. Children with anorexia may have a distorted body image, refusing to eat even when they are hungry.

2. Bulimia Nervosa: Bulimia involves repeated episodes of binge-eating followed by purging behaviors, such as vomiting or using laxatives. Children with bulimia often maintain a normal body weight and may have a preoccupation with food.

3. Binge-Eating Disorder: Binge-eating disorder involves recurrent episodes of binge-eating without purging behaviors. Children with this disorder may eat large amounts of food in a short period of time, feeling out of control during these episodes.

4. Avoidant/Restrictive Food Intake Disorder (ARFID): ARFID is characterized by a persistent lack of interest in

food or a limited range of foods consumed. This can lead to significant weight loss and malnutrition.

5. Other Specified Feeding or Eating Disorder (OSFED): This category encompasses eating disorders that do not meet the criteria for anorexia, bulimia, or binge-eating disorder. OSFED can include subthreshold forms of these disorders or unique eating behaviors, such as purging without binge-eating.

The exact causes of eating disorders in pediatric patients are not fully understood, but they are likely to be a combination of genetic, biological, and environmental factors. Certain personality traits, family dynamics, cultural pressures, and life transitions (e.g., puberty, school transitions) can increase a child's risk of developing an eating disorder.

Treatment for pediatric eating disorders usually involves a multidisciplinary approach that includes psychotherapy, nutritional counseling, and medical monitoring. Medications may be used to address comorbid conditions, such as anxiety or depression. Family involvement is critical in helping children recover from eating disorders, and early intervention can lead to better treatment outcomes.

Pediatric eating disorders are a group of psychiatric conditions characterized by abnormal eating habits and attitudes towards food and weight. Early diagnosis and treatment are crucial in preventing complications and promoting recovery. A multidisciplinary approach involving psychotherapy, nutritional counseling, and medical monitoring is often used to treat these disorders.

Autism

Autism, also known as Autism Spectrum Disorder (ASD), is a neurodevelopmental disorder that affects communication, social interaction, and behavior. It typically appears in early childhood, before the age of three, and affects boys more often than girls.

The exact cause of autism is not known, but research suggests that it may be due to a combination of genetic and environmental factors. Some studies have also suggested that abnormalities in brain development may be involved.

Children with autism may have difficulty communicating with others, both verbally and non-verbally. They may also have difficulty in making and maintaining eye contact, showing empathy, and understanding social cues such as facial expressions, gestures, and tone of voice. They may engage in repetitive behaviors or have intense interests in specific topics.

Diagnosis of autism is usually made by a team of healthcare professionals, including a pediatrician, psychologist, and speech therapist. The diagnosis is made based on observation of the child's behavior and developmental history, and may involve standardized tests and assessments.

There is no cure for autism, but early intervention with behavioral therapies and medications can help improve symptoms and enhance the child's ability to communicate and interact with others. Some of the behavioral therapies used for autism include Applied Behavior Analysis (ABA), speech therapy, and occupational therapy. Medications such as antidepressants and antipsychotics may be prescribed to help manage symptoms such as anxiety, aggression, and hyperactivity.

Post-Traumatic Stress Disorder

Post-traumatic stress disorder (PTSD) is a mental health condition that can develop in children and adolescents who have experienced or witnessed a traumatic event. Traumatic events can include physical or sexual abuse, natural disasters, accidents, violence, or sudden death of a loved one. PTSD is a serious condition that can significantly impair a child's ability to function in daily life and can have long-term effects if not properly treated.

Symptoms of PTSD can vary depending on the child's age and the nature of the traumatic event. In younger children, symptoms may include regressive behavior, bed-wetting, and separation anxiety. Older children and adolescents may experience symptoms similar to adults, including re-experiencing the traumatic event through nightmares or flashbacks, avoidance of triggers associated with the trauma, hyperarousal (e.g., difficulty sleeping or concentrating), and negative changes in mood and behavior.

Diagnosis of PTSD typically involves a comprehensive evaluation by a mental health professional, including a detailed history of the traumatic event, observation of the child's behavior and symptoms, and any necessary psychological testing. It is important for parents and caregivers to recognize the signs and symptoms of PTSD and seek professional help if they suspect their child may be affected.

Treatment of PTSD typically involves a combination of psychotherapy and medication. Cognitive-behavioral therapy (CBT) is a common form of psychotherapy that has been found to be effective in treating PTSD in children and adolescents. CBT aims to help children and their families understand and manage symptoms of PTSD, develop coping strategies, and reduce avoidance behaviors. Medications such as selective serotonin reuptake inhibitors (SSRIs) may also be prescribed to help manage symptoms of anxiety and depression.

It is important for parents and caregivers to provide a safe and supportive environment for children with PTSD. This may include seeking counseling or support groups for themselves and other family members, as well as creating a predictable and consistent routine for the child. It is also important to avoid exposing the child to triggers that may cause them to re-experience the traumatic event.

Post traumatic stress disorder is a serious mental health condition that can develop in children and adolescents who have experienced or witnessed a traumatic event. Early recognition and treatment of symptoms are important for successful recovery and long-term outcomes.

CONCLUSION

Pediatric Essentials: A Guide to Sub-specialty diagnosis highlights the intricate world of pediatric medicine. We have explored various subspecialties, delving into common diagnoses and treatments, with the aim of empowering parents and students alike.

From cardiology to neurology, pulmonology to endocrinology, each subspecialty has its unique set of challenges and approaches to care. By understanding these specialties and their roles in diagnosing and treating childhood conditions, we have equipped ourselves with the knowledge to advocate for our children's health and collaborate effectively with healthcare providers.

For parents, this book has provided valuable insights, enabling you to navigate the complexities of your child's health with confidence and clarity. It has emphasized the importance of being proactive, asking questions, and seeking second opinions when necessary. By arming yourself with knowledge, you become an active participant in your child's healthcare journey, ensuring they receive the best possible care.

To students pursuing a career in pediatrics, this book has offered a comprehensive overview, bridging the gap between theory and practice. As you continue your educational journey, we hope this book serves as a foundation for further exploration and growth in the field of pediatrics.

"Pediatric Essentials" has been carefully curated to provide concise, reliable, and practical information, respecting the valuable time and needs of our readers. By presenting key concepts in an accessible manner, we have aimed to empower and inspire, fostering collaboration and understanding between parents, students, and healthcare professionals.

As the field of pediatrics continues to evolve, new advancements, treatments, and challenges will emerge. It is essential to stay informed, updated, and engage in ongoing learning. Remember that this book serves as a starting point, providing a comprehensive overview, but it is not a substitute for professional medical advice. Always consult with trusted healthcare professionals for personalized guidance and care.

INDEX

Achondroplasia, 70,73-74

Acne, 95, 121, 231, 240-241

Acquired Immune Deficiency (AIDS), 222, 235-236, 352, 353

Acute Kidney Injury, 206, 211-212

Acute Pancreatitis, 53

Acute Poststreptococcal Glomerulonephritis, 216

Adenoiditis, 328

Adrenal Disorders, 65, 93-94

Adrenal Insufficiency, 94, 96-97

Adrenocortical Carcinoma, 94, 99-100

Alagille Syndrome, 51

Allergic dermatitis, 249

Allergic reactions, 249-250, 331, 341-342, 345-348, 354-355, 388, 395-396

Allergies, 7, 168, 238, 249-250, 271, 306, 308, 327, 331-333, 341-342, 347-350, 355, 396

Allergic rhinitis, 331, 341, 345-347

Alopecia areata, 238, 247

Alpha 1 antitrypsin Deficiency, 51

Anaphylaxis, 342, 347-348, 355-356, 388, 395-396

Amblyopia, 296, 297-298

Angioedema, 249, 396

Anxiety, 80, 101, 121, 131-132, 135, 139, 142, 252, 261-265, 269, 271, 282, 311, 320-321, 375, 410-411, 414-416, 420-422

Anorexia nervosa, 411, 419-420

Apert syndrome, 339

Apnea of prematurity, 401

Appendicitis, 387, 394

Aortic Stenosis, 16, 27-28

Arrhythmias, 10, 18, 22, 24, 26, 28, 30-32, 37, 39, 112

Astigmatism, 296, 298-301

Asthma, 6, 121, 167, 168-170, 173, 185, 335, 341-345, 349, 387-388, 395-396

Asthma exacerbation, 395-396

Attention deficit hyperactivity disorder, 7, 125, 132-134, 252, 255-257, 269, 410, 411-414

Atrial Septal Defect, 9, 11-13, 406

Autism Spectrum Disorder, 125, 134-135, 252, 253-255, 259-260, 411, 420

Autoimmune disorders, 49, 77, 96, 119, 121, 136, 158, 207, 209, 213, 216, 230, 354, 362-364

Avoidant restrictive food intake disorder, 419

Autopsy, 358, 365-367

Bedwetting, 181, 273, 279-283

Behcet's Syndrome, 193, 204-205

Biliary Atresia, 51

Binge eating disorder, 419-420

Bipolar disorder, 252, 264, 410-411, 417-418

Birth injuries, 400, 408-409

Birthmarks, 237, 241-242

Bladder exstrophy, 274, 285-277

Blocked tear duct, 297, 307-308

Bloodstream Infections, 221, 228-229

Brachial plexus injury, 408

Brain Tumors, 6, 71, 118-119, 126, 131, 132, 145, 150-152, 357

Bronchiolitis, 167, 174-176, 221-223, 388

Bronchitis, 6, 167, 172-174, 185, 335, 387

Bronchitis, Chronic, 173, 185

Bulimia nervosa, 411, 419-420

Cafe-au-lait lesions, 242

Calcium and Bone Deficiencies, 66, 106-107

Campylobacter, 56

Cancer, 6, 48, 54, 55, 60, 61, 84, 85, 94, 96, 99, 100, 106, 145-151, 162-165, 231, 242, 277, 332, 337-338, 352, 357-360,

384

Cardiomyopathy, 10, 32-33

Cardiovascular Disease, 42-43, 67, 69, 91, 106, 117, 123-124

Cataracts, congenital, 296, 301-303

Celiac Disease, 6, 44, 48-49, 62-63, 113

Cellulitis, 221, 226-227, 238, 248, 306

Cerebral palsy, 6, 125, 126, 128-130, 181, 259, 260, 368-372, 408

Charcot-Marie Tooth, 136, 377

Chest Pain, 11, 31-32, 34, 36, 38, 39-40, 41, 101, 162, 178, 190, 223, 234, 315, 389

Chlamydia, 221, 231

Choanal atresia, 332

Cholesteatoma, 329

Chronic Cough, 46, 167, 171, 184-186

Chronic Kidney Disease, 113, 206, 212-213, 287-288

Cleft lip, 328

Cleft palate, 19-20, 72, 93, 105

Coarctation, 9, 19-20, 72, 93, 105

Common cold, 169, 221, 223

Conduct disorder, 253, 265-266

Congenital Adrenal Hyperplasia, 94-95, 102

Congenital anomalies, 212, 215, 274, 285, 287, 290, 327

Congenital heart disease, 400, 405-407

Congenital Kidney Abnormalities, 206, 214-216

Conjunctivitis, 297, 306

Contact Dermatitis, 238, 249

Corneal abrasion, 297, 308-309

Craniosynostosis, 339

Croup, 223, 335, 388, 389

Cushing's Syndrome, 94, 97-99, 113, 115, 120-121

Cystic Fibrosis, 6, 44, 62, 167, 170-172, 186, 219, 310, 313-314, 331, 358

Dandruff, 238, 246-247

Dehydration, 38, 52, 62, 112, 119-120, 155, 206, 211, 217-220, 224-226, 387, 391-392

Dermatomyositis, 192, 195-197

Depression, 82-83, 116, 121, 139, 252, 271, 410-411, 415-417, 420, 422

Developmental delay, 6, 73, 82, 125, 235, 253, 268-270, 310, 320-321, 324, 339-340, 352, 369, 381-383, 398, 402, 407

Deviated septum, 327, 331

Diabetic Ketoacidosis, 67

Down syndrome, 146, 148, 181, 258, 260, 269, 310-313, 381, 406

Duplex Kidney, 215

Dyscalculia, 252, 257

Dysgraphia, 257

Dyslexia, 252, 257

Eating disorders, 253, 270-272, 411, 419-420

Eczema, 237, 238-240, 249, 342, 349-351

Encephalitis, 126, 142, 221, 229-231, 390

Epiglottitis, 334-335

Epileptic seizures, 390

Erysipelas, 248

E. coli, 221, 225-226

Eye infection, 297, 306-308

Failure to thrive, 45, 58, 188, 235, 275, 279, 324, 353, 406

Familial Adenomatous Polyposis, 60

Farsightedness, 296, 298-300

Febrile seizures, 387, 390

Folliculitis, 238, 247-248

Food allergies, 341-342, 347-349, 355, 396

Foreign body, aspiration, 336, 389

Fragile-X syndrome, 258, 269, 311, 320-321, 381

Functional Gastrointestinal Disorder, 44, 49-51

Gastroenteritis, 45, 55-56, 221, 224, 387, 394

Gastroesophageal Reflux Disorder, 44-46, 58, 185

Gastrointestinal disorders, 44, 49, 387, 393-395

Gastrointestinal Infections, 45, 55-57, 221, 224-226

Gastroparesis, 45, 58-59

General anxiety disorder, 262, 410, 414

Giardia, 56, 225

Glomerulonephritis, 206, 208-210, 216

Gonorrhea, 221, 231

Grave's Disease, 79, 86-87

Growth Disorders, 6, 65, 69-70

Growth Hormone Deficiency, 69-71, 115-117

Hashimoto's Disease, 78, 83-84

Head injuries, 131, 142, 387, 390, 392, 408

Head lice, 246

Hearing loss, 74, 79

Heart Block, Congenital, 10, 28-30

Hemangioma, 238, 241, 250-251, 328, 338

Hemolytic Anemia, 145, 158-160, 206

Hemolytic Uremic Syndrome, 206, 210-211

Hemophilia, 145, 152-153

Henoch Scholen Purpura, 193, 202-204

Hepatitis, 44, 51, 53, 158

Herpes Simplex Virus, 227, 231, 248

Hirschsprung's, 58-59

Hives, 238, 249, 342, 347-348, 353-355, 395-396

Human Immunodeficiency Virus, 235

Human Papillomavirus, 222, 231, 244-246, 248

Hydronephrosis, 215, 273-276, 283-284, 288

Hyperlipidemia, 66, 123-124

Hyperthyroidism, 78, 80-81, 84, 86-87, 113

Hypertension, 10-11, 20, 40-41, 184, 209, 215, 287

Hypoglycemia, 66-67, 121-123, 390

Hypogonadism, 45-47

Hypoplastic Left Heart, 10-13

Hypospadias, 138, 146

Hypothyroidism, 36, 70, 74-75, 78-80, 81-83, 84

Hypothyroidism, Congenital, 74-75, 78-80

IgA Neuropathy, 216

Immune Thrombocytopenia, 145, 156-158, 160-162

Immunodeficiency disorders, 342, 353

Impetigo, 216, 221, 226, 238, 248

Inguinal hernia, 274, 291-292
Influenza, 177, 223
Inherited metabolic disorders, 311, 324-325
Intellectual disability, 74, 76, 78-79, 82, 129, 252, 258-259, 310-312, 320-321, 324, 370
Interstitial Lung Disease, 168, 188-189
Intestinal Dysmotility, 45, 58-59
Intestinal Polyps, 45, 59-61
Intraventricular hemorrhage, 401
Intussusception, 394
Jaundice, 51-52, 54, 74-75, 79-80, 154, 159, 315, 399, 403-405
Juvenile Idiopathic Arthritis, 6, 60-61, 107, 110-111, 126, 192, 193
Juvenile Polyps, 60-61
Kawasaki's Disease, 10, 35-36, 192, 198-199
Keratitis, 297, 306
Kidney Stones, 112, 214-215, 218-220, 275
Klinefelter's Syndrome, 70, 77-78, 88, 102
Labial adhesions, 274, 294-295
Lactose Intolerance, 45, 62-63, 259-261
Language disorder, 252, 257
Laryngitis, 333
Laryngomalacia, 328, 336
Learning Disability, 76-77, 129, 252, 256-259, 312, 320-321, 324
Leukemia, 6, 145, 146-148, 312, 357
Lipid Disorders, 11, 42-43
Liver Disease, 44, 51-53, 171, 352
Lymphoma, 6, 145, 148-150, 337, 357
Lupus Nephritis, 216
Lyme Disease, 222, 232-234
Malabsorption, 44-45, 61-64
Malrotation, 394
Meningitis, 126, 142, 221, 229-231, 390, 400
Metabolic disorders, 32, 65-66, 68, 126-127, 302, 311, 324-325, 358, 364-365, 390

Migraines, 125-126, 131, 140-142
Mongolian spot, 242
Mood disorder, 98, 252, 261-265, 410
Motility Disorder, 45-46, 57-59
Multicystic Dysplastic Kidney Disease, 215, 287
Muscular Dystrophy, 125, 136-138, 310, 316-318, 368, 376
Myasthenia Gravis, 136, 368-369
Myopathies, Congénital, 136
Nasal congestion, 181, 185, 330-332, 345-346
Nasal polyps, 313, 330-331
Nearsightedness, 296, 298-300
Necrotizing enterocolitis, 394, 401
Neonatal abstinence syndrome, 400, 407
Nephritis, 207, 216-217
Nephrotic Syndrome, 206, 207-208
Neuroblastoma, 146, 162-164, 338
Neurofibromatosis, 150, 242, 310-311, 318-320
Neurogenic bladder, 275
Neuropathy, 67-68
Norovirus, 55, 225
Obstructive uropathy, 207, 288
Organ dysfunction, 202
Otitis externa, 328-329
Otitis media, 328
Pancreatic Cysts, 14
Pancreatic Disease, 44, 53-55
Pancreatitis, Chronic, 53-54
Patent Ductus Arteriosus, 9, 14-15, 406
Penile adhesions, 274, 292-293
Peutz Jeghers Syndrome, 60-61
Pharyngitis, 333
Pheochromocytoma, 94, 100-101
Phimosis, 274, 289-290
Pierre Robin syndrome, 340
Pigmented birthmark, 237, 241-242
Pituitary Disorders, 66, 114-116

Pneumonia, 167, 177-180, 221-224, 230, 236, 353, 387-400, 403

Poisoning, 45, 56, 225, 388, 396-398

Polycystic Kidney Disease, 215, 288

Port wine stain, 241

Post traumatic stress disorder, 411, 421-423

Postnasal Drip, 185

Prader-Willi Syndrome, 70, 75-76

Precocious Puberty, 87, 88-89, 95, 115, 117-118

Prematurity, 128, 228, 269, 303-304, 369, 399-402

Pruritus, 250

Psoriasis, 237-238, 242-244

Ptosis, 296, 304-306

Puberty Disorders, 65, 70-71, 87-93

Pulmonary Hypertension, 10, 36-37, 184

Pulmonary Stenosis, 10, 25-27

Reactive Arthritis, 192, 200-201

Renal Agenesis, 214-215, 287

Renal Tubular Acidosis, 207, 217-218

Respiratory distress, 168, 183-184, 186-188, 228, 342-343, 387, 388-389, 399

Respiratory Distress Syndrome, 168, 186-187, 399, 401, 402-403, 405

Retinopathy of prematurity, 296, 303-304, 401

Rhabdomyosarcoma, 338

Rheumatic Fever, 10, 33-34

Ringworm, 221, 227, 247

Rotavirus, 55, 221, 225

Refractive error, 296-299, 300-301, 302

Renal Tubular Acidosis, 207, 217-218

Respiratory Infections, 169, 171-179, 183-186, 188-189, 221-224, 312, 343-344, 387, 401

Rotavirus, 55, 221, 225

Salivary gland tumors, 337

Salmon patch, 242

Salmonella, 56, 221, 225-226

Scabies, 227, 248

Scalp psoriasis, 237-238

Scleroderma, 192, 197-198

Seborrheic Dermatitis, 247, 249

Seizures, 126-128, 143, 324, 375, 387, 389-391

Separation anxiety disorder, 262, 410, 414, 416, 422

Sepsis, 179-180, 401

Sex, Disorders of, 65-66, 87-91, 101-106

Sexually Transmitted Infections, 222, 231-232

Short Bowel Syndrome, 45, 62

Shoulder dystocia, 408

Sickle Cell Anemia, 142, 145, 154-156, 158, 310, 314-316

Sinusitis, 327, 331-332

Skin Infections, 221, 226-228

Specific phobias, 262, 414

Spina bifida, 368-369, 372-374, 384

Sleep Apnea, 73, 167, 180-183

Social anxiety disorder, 262, 311, 410, 414

Sore throat, 46, 222-223, 332-333

Speech disorder, 259-261

Spinal cord injury, 369, 383-386

Sports injuries, 368, 374, 376, 378-381, 384, 387, 392-393

Stork bite, 242

Strabismus, 296, 298-300

Strawberry hemangioma, 241

Stroke, 126, 142-144

Stye, 306

Syncope, 10, 37-39

Syphilis, 231

Systemic Onset Juvenile Rheumatoid Arthritis, 199-200

Systemic Lupus Erythematosus, 192, 194-195, 216

Tetralogy of Fallot, 9, 16-18, 406

Thrombocytopenia, 145, 156-158, 160-162

Thyroid Disorders, 65, 70, 78-87

Thyroid Nodules, 84-85

Tinea capitis, 247

Tinnitus, 330
Tonsillitis, 328, 332-333
Tourette Syndrome, 126, 138-140, 253, 267-268
Tracheomalacia, 168, 189-191, 336
Traumatic brain injury, 126, 368, 374-376, 379
Traumatic injuries, 128, 227, 378-381, 387-388, 392-393
Treacher collins syndrome, 340
Tuberculosis, 222, 234-236
Turner Syndrome, 70, 71-73, 88, 92-93, 102, 104-105, 311, 322-323, 406
Tympanic membrane perforation, 329
Type 1 Diabetes Mellitus, 65, 66-68
Type 2 Diabetes Mellitus, 65, 68-69, 77
Undescended testes, 103, 273, 276-278
Ureteropelvic Junction Obstruction, 275, 283-285
Urinary Tract Infection, 7, 206, 213-214, 273, 276, 278-280, 282, 284, 286, 288, 294
Urticaria, 238, 249, 342, 353, 396,
Varicella Zoster, 248-249
Vascular birthmarks, 237, 241-242
Vascular malformation, 328
Vasculitis, 193, 201-205
Ventral Septal Defect, 9, 13-14, 16, 406
Vertigo, 327
Vesicoureteral reflux, 273, 275-276, 278, 280-281, 288
Vocal cord nodules, 334
Warts, 221, 231, 237, 244-246, 248
Wilm's Tumor, 164-166
Wilson's Disease, 52